HAIR TISSUE MI

An introduction for practitioners to the new technique of medical assessment which promises to have far-reaching implications in biomedicine.

HAIR TISSUE MINERAL ANALYSIS

An Emergent Diagnostic Technique

by

Jeffrey Bland
PhD

THORSONS PUBLISHERS INC.
New York

Thorsons Publishers Inc.
377 Park Avenue South
New York, New York 10016

First U.S. Edition 1984

Originally published by
Northwest Diagnostic Services, Bellevue, Washington 98007

Library of Congress Cataloging in Publication Data

Bland, Jeffrey, 1946-
Hair tissue mineral analysis.

Bibliography: p.
Includes index.
1. Hair manifestations of general diseases. 2. Hair—Analysis.
3. Trace elements—Diagnostic use. I. Title.
[DNLM: 1. Hair—Analysis. 2. Minerals—Analysis.
WR 450 B642h]
RC73.7.B58 1984 616.07'56 83-24303
ISBN 0-7225-0876-X

Printed and bound in Great Britain

Thorsons Publishers Inc. are distributed to the trade by
Inner Traditions International Ltd., New York

CONTENTS

INTRODUCTION

The use of the clinical laboratory in medical diagnosis has increased considerably over the past twenty years. The direction and emphasis of research in this area is toward the development of new methodologies which allow the early-on assessment of metabolic trends, which may if ultimately untreated result in a crisis disease sometime in the future. This approach toward health has been commonly dubbed preventive medicine, and there is considerable evidence to suggest that it may be the only cost-efficient way to approach health care in the future.[1,2]

One diagnostic technique utilized in preventive medicine which has received considerable discussion during the past ten years, and which is still considered somewhat avant-garde and suspicious, is the technique called trace mineral analysis of human hair tissue. In this technique a small amount (approximately one gram) of the patient's hair is taken from the suboccipital region of the scalp, the first inch of growth from the scalp, digested in acid or some suitable medium, and then analysed by either atomic absorption spectrophotometry, or plasma jet spectrophotometry for the presence of trace amounts of both the essential and toxic mineral elements in the hair.

In the past few years it has become clear that trace mineral nutrition and trace mineral metabolism play a significant role in maintenance of human health[3], and that in biomedicine the implications of trace mineral nutriture today are somewhat analogous to the explosion of information which occurred with regard to vitamin nutriture in the 1920s and 1930s.

As we learn more about the important role that these trace elements play in human health it becomes obvious that there is a great need for sensitive, convenient and inexpensive methods for screening patients for their trace element status.

Recently Maugh, has suggested that hair mineral analysis has the potential to become a remarkable tool to complement blood, serum and urine mineral analysis in assessing mineral status.[4] He points out that hair is easily collected without trauma on the part of the donor, it can be stored without deterioration, and its contents can be analysed relatively easily. Trace elements, he points out, are accumulated in the hair at concentrations that are generally at least ten times higher than those present in blood, serum or urine, and may provide a continuous record of nutritional status and exposure to heavy metal pollutants such as cadmium, lead, mercury and arsenic.

Most research has focussed on the measurement of metallic element concentrations within human hair tissue in hopes of early recognition of nutritional deficiencies or elucidating certain pathophysiologies which have relationships to mineral status. Members of the first transition series of elements, including chromium, copper and zinc, have received the most study, with less work having been done on the alkaline metals such as sodium and potassium and alkaline earths such as magnesium and calcium. The toxic element family has been investigated to a great degree, with representative examples being lead, mercury, cadmium, and now aluminium, receiving more attention. Hair element concentrations of all these examples have been related to the systemic status of the donor.

The function and chemical form of the elements in hair filaments remain obscure; apparently, these elements are incorporated into the filament as it is synthesized in the follicle and therefore may more represent intracellular levels of elements than extracellular concentrations. Follicles exposed to a large amount of a particular element incorporate a large amount of it into the growing hair protein matrix. As Klevay points out, 'Analysis of human hair is an experimental technique that has clinical promise . . . . The usefulness of the method will grow as more of the factors that influence the concentration of metallic elements in hair are identified.'[5]

Recently standarization methods for the analysis of ultratrace elements in hair have been promulgated, and analytical procedures have been codified, and the clinical implications of these results have become better understood by health scientists. This book reviews recent contemporary literature as it relates to the strengths and weaknesses of the hair trace element technique in assessing mineral status for both toxic mineral exposure and essential trace element sufficiency.

1.

CRITICISMS OF HAIR TISSUE MINERAL ANALYSIS

In the face of all the encouraging information concerning the potential clinical utility of hair mineral analysis, there still remains a very considered controversy surrounding its potential routine application in health screening. Dr Paul Lazar has pointed out in a paper putting forward the position of the American Medical Association that 'In selected applications in forensic, clinical or epidemiologic medicine, trace metal hair analysis, along with other tests, is a useful tool. Nevertheless, present scientific knowledge does not support the use of metal levels in hair for broad, sophisticated, subtle diagnostic purposes . . . and certainly hair analysis is not desirable for routine use.'[1]

Lazar challenges the utility of hair element testing as a screening tool for element status on the basis of six considerations, which include:

1. The variation in hair trace mineral content is related to differing hair colours and beauty treatments.
2. Changes in the hair trace element levels may occur as the result of differing washing procedures.
3. Environmental perturbations, such as aerosols and fall-out, as well as constitutents of hard water, may influence mineral levels of hair.
4. There is no relationship between hair trace mineral levels and a tissue level of the mineral in question, or a specific pathophysiological process.
5. The variation in mineral levels may relate to the position on the scalp from which the sample was taken.
6. Variations in quality control of the analytical laboratories or technique used to determine the levels of trace elements in hair, including the lack of standard procedures within the industry, may result in no uniformity of values.

Each of these topics needs to be discussed and evaluated to assess the utility of hair element testing as a health appraisal technique.

On reflection upon the criticisms it should be recalled that the article by Dr Lazar was published in 1974, meaning that the references used in deriving the conclusions in the article were taken from information pre-1974. In the past nine years a virtual explosion of information has appeared in the world's peer-group reviewed literature surrounding trace mineral analysis and more specifically the use of hair tissue as a diagnostic tool for assessing trace mineral nutriture adequacies. It is with these new pieces of information available that we need reflect, then, upon the six criticisms raised in the original critique of the hair mineral analysis technique. The following discussion is designed to explore the six criticisms mentioned above in the light of the newly available information from our laboratory and others working in this field.

Hair Colours and Hair Treatments as they influence Hair Minerals

Evaluation of the relationship between hair colour and trace element levels was accomplished in our laboratory when we examined 3,564 hair element analyses of individuals who had a variety of hair colours and categorized the trace element composition of their hair as it related to their hair colour. In Figure 1 the results of this study are presented. In general there is no significant relationship between hair colour and trace element level, and the variation from hair colour to hair colour is not important except for the case of black-haired individuals, where there is a much higher level of hair lead. This was due to contamination of some of the samples of patients with black hair who had been using lead-containing hair colouring agents or anti-greying agents which were not screened out of the sample. Other than this curious variation there is no suggestion that hair colour is a major determinant of trace element concentrations. This perspective was supported by Chittleborough in his recent review of the analysis of human hair for trace elements.[2]

The effect that hair treatments have upon trace element analysis has been examined by Joan McKenzie. She has determined that bleaching of the hair and cold waving of the hair both have an impact upon the concentrations of the trace elements zinc and copper, but that dyeing, hair sprays, and shampoos that do not contain trace elements have little to no impact upon hair element concentration.[3]

HAIR COLOUR VERSUS MINERAL LEVELS
(All Values in mg%)

Hair Colour:	**Blonde**	**Black**	**Brown**	**Red**	**Grey**
Element					
Ca	153.0	124.0	128.0	153.0	77.0
Mg	13.5	12.9	12.6	16.7	10.1
Na	17.0	19.7	18.4	21.0	18.7
K	4.5	6.7	5.1	5.4	5.4
Cu	3.2	2.7	2.9	2.7	1.8
Fe	2.0	2.2	2.2	2.0	2.2
Zn	15.7	18.0	17.7	17.3	16.1
Mn	0.1	0.1	0.1	0.1	0.1
Cr	0.1	0.4	0.1	0.1	0.1
Se	0.30	0.2	0.2	0.2	0.2
Pb	1.3	3.2	2.2	1.7	1.9
As	0.2	0.2	0.2	0.2	0.3
Cd	0.1	0.1	0.1	0.1	0.1
Hg	0.2	0.2	0.2	0.2	0.2
Al	1.3	1.4	1.3	1.2	1.1
Number in population	423	296	2229	135	457
% males	36	49	40	37	23
% females	64	51	60	77	63

Figure 1

Influence of Washing Procedures on Hair Minerals.
A question commonly asked by those who have had occasion to explore the usefulness of human hair trace mineral analysis has been what influence the washing procedures have upon trace elements in the hair. Again, McKenzie[4] has had occasion to examine the influence of various washing procedures.

She has also determined that washing of the hair on a routine basis with aqueous wash, or in the laboratory situation with non-aqueous solvent, such as heptane or hexane followed by an aqueous wash, will remove the absorbed elements, leaving behind only the intracellular bound elements which were presumably deposited during protein synthesis and more reflect systemic levels of the element than environmental contaminants. Recently washing curves have been generated for a number of the elements and it was found that after the second aqueous wash the level of element in the hair remained constant throughout any additional washings, suggesting that the endogenously bound elements are tightly retained and not easily removed by repetitive aqueous washings[5]. The shape of a representative washing curve is as seen in Figure 2.

REPRESENTATIVE WASHING CURVE FOR
HAIR TRACE ELEMENTS
(taken from Salmela, Ref. 28)

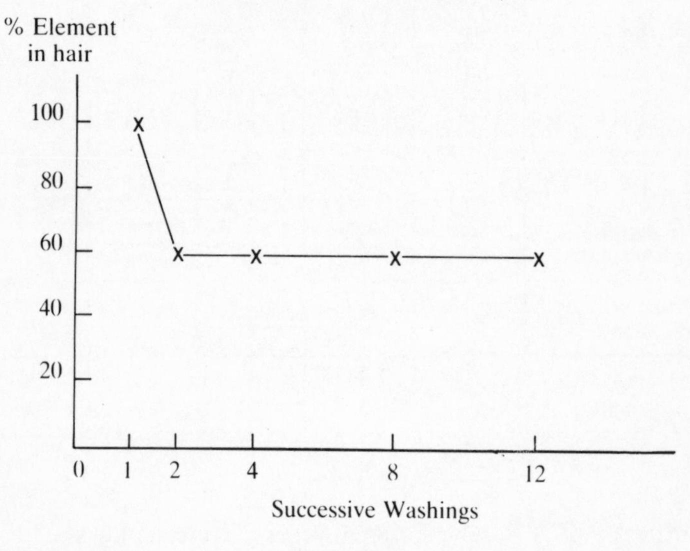

Figure 2

In Figure 3 you will note the influence of various washing procedures on human hair which has been soaked in solutions containing zinc or copper of either low or high concentration, as it relates to a control hair sample. You will note that in the washing procedures utilizing non-ionic detergent plus EDTA* it has been found that even when soaking the hair in 100 mcg of zinc per millilitre the washing procedure reduces the concentration upon analysis to that of

*ethylenediaminetetraacetic acid

the control level. This same phenomenon is seen in the copper-treated hair at the low concentration, but not at the high concentration, where even the best washing procedure cannot reduce the copper concentration of the hair lower than 214 parts per million, whereas the control is 51.8 parts per million. This would indicate that individuals who have been exposed to exogenous sources of zinc, such as found as zinc pyrithione in some shampoos, may have this exogenous zinc contaminant removed by appropriate washing procedures utilized by the analytical laboratory, whereas those individuals who routinely swim in chlorinated swimming pools which contain high levels of copper, will have their hair contaminated with copper even under the best of washing procedures, due to the tenacity of copper binding to the hair and the inability of the washing procedure to remove these high levels of copper.

EFFECT OF WASHING PROCEDURES

Washing Procedure	**Zn μg/g**			**Cu μg/g**		
	Treatment			**Treatment**		
	Control	**100 μg Zn/ml**	**1 μg Zn/ml**	**Control**	**50 μg Cu/ml**	**0.1 μg Cu/ml**
Not washed	228	407	270	61.7	1598	70.4
Ionic detergent	215	383	236	56.5	1425	70.7
Nonionic detergent	191	288	197	55.5	414	67.8
EDTA	198	255	192	59.2	273	59.7
Ionic detergent + EDTA	196	283	217	53.2	346	63.4
Nonionic detergent + EDTA	184	247	183	51.8	214	57.7

Figure 3

From these data, then, one can see that in washing of the hair previous to analysis a hydrocarbon solvent, followed by an aqueous wash, that, many of the exogenous elements are removed, thereby leaving behind only the endogenous elements which are deposited by synthesis at the hair follicle, presumably as a result of incorporation from the arterial blood supply. This point is reinforced in an elegant series of experiments done by Kennington[4].

In this study hair was soaked in a radioactive sodium solution for ten days and then the amount of radioactivity which was incorporated was counted. This hair was then washed with water and the radioactivity checked. It was found that extensive washing with water would ultimately remove almost all of the radioactive sodium which was deposited in the hair by soaking. This hair after washing, then, was activated in a neutron flux, so that any residual sodium which was present in the hair initially, and not incorporated as radioactive sodium, would be activated to a different type of sodium, sodium 24.

The original hair was also washed with water and also equally activated in a neutron flux, and the hair after having been exposed to the radioactive sodium 22 solution, washed with water and then activated with the neutron flux, was compared in activity to the original hair which was just washed with water and then activated. This scheme is outlined in Figure 4.

It was found in comparison of the sodium 24 activities of both the control hair and the treated hair that their activities were very similar. The conclusion of the author was, then, that there are two forms of an element found in hair: one form is washed out with relative ease and is basically bound to the surface and presumably is exogenously deposited, whereas the other remains fixed and is at about the same level after extensive washing. Presumably, then, it is a result of deposition during hair protein synthesis and reflects systemic levels of the element and not exogenous contaminants.

This is a very important conclusion when taken in conjunction with McKenzie's work. It indicates that the hair, when exposed to exogenous contaminants such as lead, mercury, chromium, or zinc can have these contaminating elements removed by the appropriate washing procedures. This washing procedure, however, will not remove the internally bound trace elements which are those which have been deposited at the hair follicle site in synthesis, and presumably reflect more systemic levels of an element in question and not the exogenous contaminants.

For those individuals attempting to utilize trace element analysis of human hair tissue as a view of systemic trace element flux, it is important to recognize this differentiation.

LINEAR REGRESSION OF HAIR COPPER VERSUS
COPPER IN UNWASHED LIVER

G.S. Kennington, *Science, 155* (1967), 588.

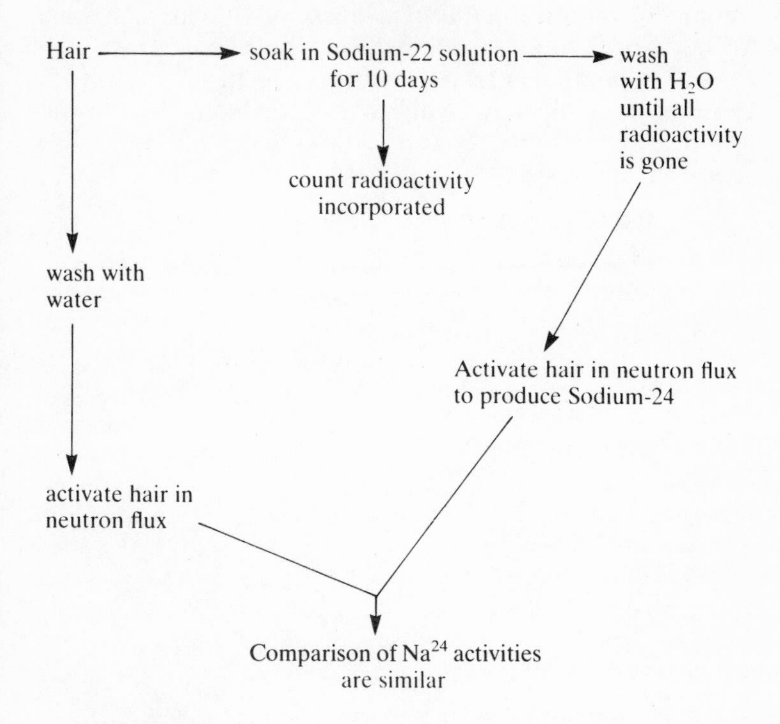

Conclusions:
Two forms of an element: one washed out with relative ease and bound to the surface, and the other fixed and remains at about the same level after extensive washing, presumably deposited during hair protein synthesis.

Figure 4

One is not concerned in this case about the total levels of trace element in question, but rather the levels of trace elements in that specific hair sample which result from metabolic deposition. The previous studies indicate clearly that, even in the case of an element as easily solubilized as sodium, which would presumably be the most easily washed out element of all of those routinely analyzed, the endogenously deposited form of the element is very tenaciously bound to the hair protein matrix and is not easily leached out even after extensive washing.

It has been found in our laboratory that washing of a hair sample for several months in distilled water leads to virtually no additional loss of sodium from the hair after the first three five-minute water washes. This again re-confirms the fact that those elements which are deposited by hair protein synthesis are firmly bound to the hair and not easily removed by washing procedures.

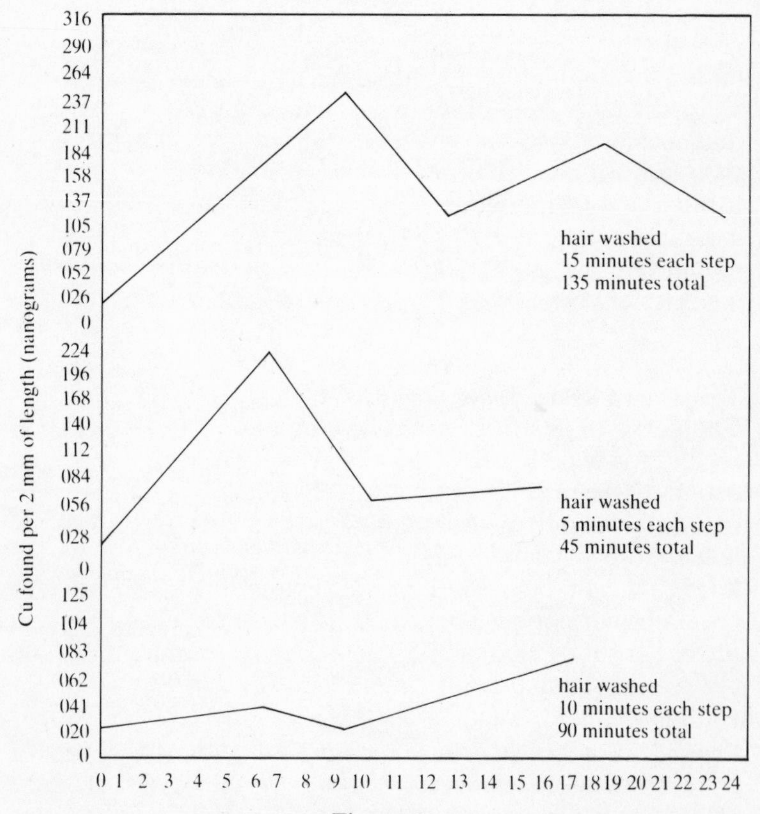

Figure 5

Inspection of Figure 5 once again reinforces this point. It can be seen from the work of Pate et al[6] that washing up to 135 minutes removes virtually no more of the element copper from the hair then washing 45 minutes, if the sample is procured from the first 5 centimeters from the scalp. As one goes to longer hair lengths (greater than three inches from the scalp) it can be seen that the hair picks up considerable more exogenous contaminants, presumably because the hair protein unwinds and becomes more porous and permeable to exogenous contaminants.

These data indicate that one must procure the hair from the first inch of growth from the scalp, which is the last three months on the average of hair growth, for the element analysis in question to be reflective of systemic levels of that particular element. It has also been found that hairs which are contiguous to one another on the scalp can have reasonably varied trace element concentrations. It is only by taking several hundred hairs at the suboccipital region of the scalp that one gets an average value of trace minerals in human hair tissue for that particular patient, which allows then a more general appraisal of trace mineral metabolism for that unique individual. The use of very small hair sample sizes or single hairs is in considerable question when attempting to utilize this data for answering questions concerning trace mineral metabolism or nutriture for that patient[6].

Tissue and Hair Trace Mineral Levels

The question as to whether trace mineral analysis of hair is related to tissue levels of the mineral in question have been explored recently by Klevay et al. Inspection of Figure 6 shows the result of the examination of hair tissue copper levels from particular animals to that of their liver copper levels. It can be seen that there is a linear correlation between hair copper levels and liver copper levels, both in the microsomal and whole unwashed liver fractions. The correlation is statistically significant at the 99.9 per cent confidence limits, and it can be seen that as hair copper increases there is a monotonic increase in liver copper. This is an excellent example of the relationship between system wet tissue levels of a particular essential trace element and its level of deposition in the hair tissue.

This is an exciting result in that liver biopsy work for a particular element in question is considerably more difficult and invasive than the procurement of a trace mineral hair

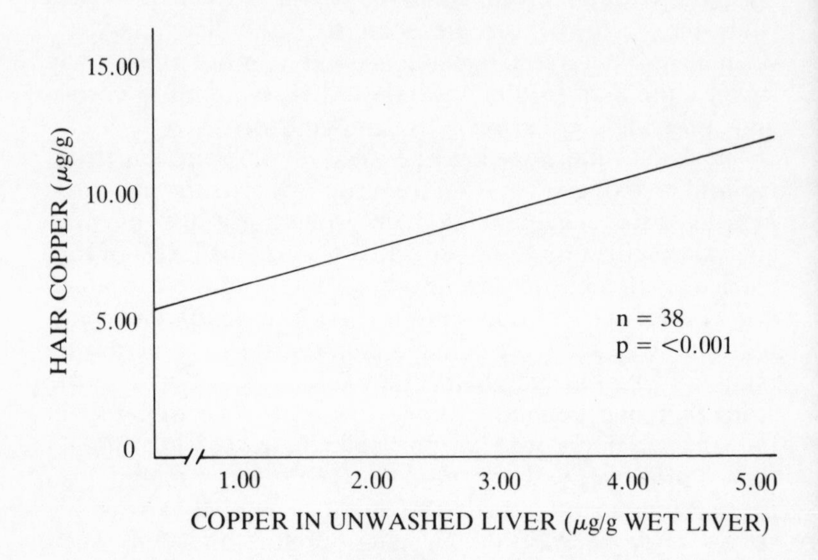

Figure 6

tissue specimen. The liver copper-containing metalloenzymes, which are involved in drug detoxification and the liver mixed microsomal oxidase family of enzymes, are extremely important in catabolizing many materials which could elicit long-term toxic effects if they were not oxidized and broken down. Insufficiencies of mixed microsomal enzyme function in the liver are in part related to insufficiencies of copper at the microsomal site.

The use of hair trace mineral analysis, then, may be of considerable importance in relating the drug detoxification system and hepatic oxidase enzyme function to that of a readily obtainable and easily analysable hair tissue source. These data do not confirm the fact that all trace elements in hair are directly related to tissue levels within specific organ systems, but it does certainly raise the question as to the general applicability of wet tissue trace element concentration as it relates to the elements concentrations in human hair.

Hair trace elements are tightly bound by the supporting

protein matrix keratin, which is rich in sulfhydryl amino acids, providing the sulfhydryl group as a strong chelating ligand to bind heavy elements available. Recently, much more research has been done on the levels of trace elements in hair and their correlation with tissue levels or pathophysiological processes in the body. As indicated Klevay reported that elevated hair copper levels were associated with liver copper elevations.[7] More recent work indicates that hair zinc and chromium levels are reflective of certain aspects of immune status and glucose tolerance, respectively.[8,9]

Recent applications of hair element testing during pregnancy indicate that hair may have significant potential value in assessing aspects of maternal trace element status throughout pregnancy and of trace element sufficiency in infancy.[10,11]

Hair trace element concentrations do not always correlate with serum element levels. This results due to the differences between the status of the element in serum and in hair. First, serum analysis is a measure of the extracellular levels of an element which may not represent intracellular tissue deposits of a specific element, but rather reflects an equilibrium of an extracellular pool of an element, which is but a small amount of the total body content of that element. Hair element status is more reflective of intracellular element concentrations and potentially of aspects of body pool dynamics.

Secondly, contamination or alterations in trace element level of the serum may occur as it relates to venapuncture. Temporary venous occlusion which occurs when blood is drawn has recently been shown to cause alteration in trace element concentrations of plasma.[12] It has also been found that vacutainer tube stoppers may lead to contamination of serum samples with zinc, in that zinc is contained in the rubber stoppers.[13]

It should be pointed out that hair trace element levels are not solely reflective of levels of an element that have been ingested in the diet, but rather are reflective of the complex process of ingestion, absorption, and deposition in a growing hair protein.

As Gershoff has pointed out, the total diet and physiological status of the individual can influence the level of trace elements in the hair and interpretation of patterns of elements in hair should take into account these known interrelationships.[14]

Dietary Influences on Hair Minerals

Another question which is commonly asked with regard to the use of hair trace mineral analyses is whether the levels of the trace element in hair are in fact reflective only of the levels of ingestion of that particular element, or whether the levels of that element in hair are reflective of other factors, which may then influence its appearance in the hair. The work of Gershoff et al[1'] clearly indicates that the latter is the case. Inspection of Figure 7 indicates the results of feeding rats diets which have identical levels of trace

EFFECTS OF DIETS VARYING IN VITAMINS, PROTEIN, AND CARBOHYDRATE, BUT NOT MINERALS, ON RAT HAIR CATION LEVELS.

Diet	Wt gain/ 12 wk	Zn	Mg	Cu
1, low vitamins	190 ± 8	257 ± 28	69 ± 5	21 ± 3
2, low B vitamins	254 ± 10	182 ± 17	69 ± 5	15 ± 2
3, low vitamins A and D	244 ± 4	163 ± 24	62 ± 4	8 ± 1
4,	309 ± 15	122 ± 29	62 ± 2	8 ± 2
5, low vitamins, no gelatin	120 ± 10	128 ± 6	56 ± 3	10 ± 2
6, low vitamins, no gelatin, 16.5% casein	212 ± 13	150 ± 11	48 ± 4	10 ± 2
7, low vitamins, 55.3% sucrose	206 ± 18	155 ± 17	53 ± 8	9 ± 1
8, 55.3% sucrose	342 ± 7	96 ± 11	57 ± 6	12 ± 4

Unless otherwise stated diets contain 10.5% casein, 6% gelatin, 49% lactose, and adequate vitamins.

Figure 7

elements, but which vary in the levels of vitamins, proteins, and carbohydrates. One can see by inspection of these data that the levels of elements deposited in hair vary widely, depending upon the particular macro- and micronutrients which are found in the diet in conjunction with these trace elements. For instance, it is noticed that on the diet where 55 per cent of the calories come as sucrose the level of zinc in the hair is 9.6mg per cent, whereas the diet containing 16.5 per cent of the calories as casein (a milk protein) the level of zinc is 15mg per cent, both diets containing equal amounts of zinc.

It is therefore clear that the full complement of the diet can influence the levels of trace elements deposited ultimately in hair, as well as other systemic and metabolic influences. The amount of a nutrient ultimately finding itself in cellular function is only partly related to the amount ingested. It should be recalled that the nutrient in question must be appropriately digested and absorbed, distributed, taken up by the cell by membrane transport, and ultimately utilized at the cellular site for appropriate presence of that nutrient to be felt.

One can see, then, that the use of trace mineral element analysis of hair is more than just assessment of the mineral ingestion of a particular patient, but rather a reflection on the total metabolic consequence of trace elements in that individual patient as it relates to their macronutrients (protein, carbohydrate and fat) and micronutrients (water, fat-soluble vitamins and other mineral intakes) and hormonal status. This point is clearly substantiated by the work of Greger et al, in which he looked at the nutritional status of adolescent girls, with regard to zinc, copper and iron, and the relationship then to these elements in the hair.[15] Greger found that the mean concentration of zinc in 183 hair samples in the autumn was 21.6 ± 6.4mg per cent, whereas in the spring the mean concentration of zinc in 176 hair samples was 19.1 ± 3.6mg per cent. When comparing the hair zinc mineral levels to the serum levels measured on the same subjects it was revealed that zinc levels in the hair and serum samples were inversely correlated ($R = -0.267$, $P<0.012$).

The conclusions that these authors derive are that the observations suggest that neither of the parameters — serum zinc or hair zinc — is the ideal way to measure zinc nutritional status. Hair zinc represents zinc nutritional status of subject at an earlier time when the hair was formed, whereas serum zinc levels represent a combination of factors besides diet affecting blood zinc levels when the sample was collected. It may be suggested then that a combination of serum and hair trace mineral levels might give the best diagnostic information about the state of trace mineral nutriture and metabolism of an individual patient.

Additional work from this study found that hair copper levels, but not serum copper levels, were significantly correlated to hematocrit levels ($R = 0.267$, $P < 0.009$). Again, these results suggest strongly that there is a relationship between trace mineral metabolism and trace mineral nutriture and the levels of that respective element in the hair tissue. The relationship is obviously not direct, but rather one that reflects many different perturbing parameters including absorption and the presence and absence of other nutrients and metabolic fitness.

To dismiss, however, the validity of this technique on the basis of this confusion would be to lose much useful potential diagnostic information. The confusion results from our lack of familiarity with this technique and ability to use this very meaningful data in a manner that reflects greater clinical experience.

Two pieces of work that confirm the usefulness of the hair trace mineral technique in determining relative trace mineral metabolic or nutritional imbalances are found in the work of Hambidge[16] and Erten et al.[17] Utilizing Denver Head Start pre-school children, Hambidge, by dietary recall studies, was able to find that low-income diets provide relatively little zinc. It was found that the mean hair zinc concentration was 8.7mg per cent, and the mean plasma zinc concentration 74.5mcg/100 ml. These levels were both lower ($P < 0.005$) than those of middle-income children of similar age. Sixty-eight per cent of the Head Start study group had hair zinc concentration less than 7mg per cent and/or a plasma zinc concentration of less than 68mcg/100 ml, which indicates that inadequate zinc nutrition may be common among pre-school children with low growth percentiles from low-income families.

This study is of great significance with regard to the diagnostic usefulness of hair trace mineral levels in that it clearly illustrates that children who have the clinical manifestations of zinc deficiency are found to have with very great diagnostic correlation low hair zinc levels. This study was further expanded by work done in Turkey by Erten et al[17], in which the hair zinc levels of 115 health subjects (50 girls and 65 boys between the ages of 0 to 15 years) were determined. It was found in their study that the levels of hair zinc increased as a function of age and there were no specifically significant differences with regard to sex or colour of the hair, as we have seen in the previous work described earlier. In a protein-calorie malnourished group it was found that the hair zinc levels were significantly different from a group of healthy subjects of the same age range.

The Relationship Between Serum and Hair Mineral Levels
In conclusion, it can be said that there is still confusion as to the direct relationship between serum levels of a trace element and the hair levels of that element in question. However, the diagnostic usefulness of serum and hair measurement when taken together is clear with regard to the ascertaining of unique trace mineral metabolic imbalances, which may present themselves clinically as discreet physiological inadequacies, such as the growth retardation observed by Hambidge in the Head Start school children who were zinc deficient.

In an unpublished study we have recently found that in patients presenting themselves with zinc deficiencies such as

SERUM ZINC AND HAIR ZINC
in Patients Showing Clinical Symptoms of Zinc Deficiency

Symptom: white spots under fingernails, eczema, poor appetite, dysmenorrhea.

Number: 6 patients

Before Therapy

Hair Zinc level	32 ± 6 mg%
Serum Zinc	64 ± 6 μg/100 ml.

After 24 mg. oral zinc/day Therapy (Retest after 90 days)

Hair Zinc level	22 ± 2 mg%
Serum Zinc	110 ± 30 μg/100 ml.

Clinical Note: Symptoms were markedly improved after therapy.

Figure 8

white spots under the fingernails, eczema, poor appetite, and dysmenorrhea there may be found in these individuals an elevated hair zinc level. Inspection of Figure 8 reveals this particular relationship. Six patients who presented themselves with these zinc deficiency symptoms had elevated hair zinc levels at the onset of zinc therapy and suboptimal serum zinc levels. After 24mg of oral zinc per day for three months, their clinical symptoms were alleviated, their hair zinc levels had gone down within normal range and their serum zinc levels had gone up into normal range. This again is another clear example of the complex relationship between hair trace mineral levels and serum levels of an element in question. One can see easily why hair trace mineral diagnostic usefulness may have received a bad reputation in the past in that there is no clear linear relationship between the levels in hair and the levels in serum, and there may very well be a differing metabolic partition effect that is explored with hair trace mineral levels than that which is explored with serum trace mineral levels. Whereas serum levels are looking at the level of a trace element extracellularly, the hair trace mineral levels may be looking at intracellular trace element concentrations, which are particularly concentrated in the tissue that is highest in chelating amino acids such as cystine, of which hair is the unique representative example.

One, then, might expect there to be considerable differences between the information derived from serum levels of a trace element and the levels in hair. Hair tissue levels may more adequately reflect intracellular element concentrations whereas serum levels may better reflect membrane transport and extracellular phenomena.

Laker has recently reviewed the potential methodologies that are available for assessing essential trace element and toxic element exposure which include blood, urine, hair, teeth, and nails. He goes on to point out that three of these can be discounted for general use: urine which gives information only on what the body has lost, not on what is retained; teeth which are rarely used, because they are not readily available; and nails, of which there is little known about the trace element concentrations. Two possibilities are then left: blood and hair.[18]

The two methods reflect body trace element status over different scales of time. Trace element concentrations in blood are transient related to the supply of elements in the previous hours or days, whereas hair element levels provide a lasting record of levels of exposure over the past few months. Laker points out that for elements such as the toxic heavy metals, where cumulative intake and exposure information are desired, blood reveals little and hair element concentrations provide much more information. Petering, et al, concluded that 'blood is not a suitable material to analyze for cadmium since the metal remains in the blood for only a very brief period and in consequence the levels are always extremely low'.[19] In an Italian study, blood was found to be a less reliable index of exposure to mercury than hair tissue.[20] Blood has been found to be a very complex biological sample from which trace element data are difficult to extract due to its heterogeneous composition. Whole blood, plasma, serum, leucocytes, or erythrocytes each exhibit different concentrations of the trace elements. With blood, trace elements are being transferred from one component to another in constant dynamics and therefore the analysis of a serum sample at one moment may change on reanalysis at a time not too far distant.

Hambidge and Mertz have pointed out that blood is of little help in determining chromium, copper, and selenium status, and other elements may also be inadequately represented by blood analysis.[21,22]

As pointed out by Laker, given these problems with blood trace element analysis, hair deserves serious consideration as an alternative biopsy specimen for element status, in that it offers the following advantages:[18]

1. Hair provides a better assessment of long-term exposure to trace elements because short-term variations are averaged out.
2. Unlike blood, hair is an inert and chemically homogeneous substance which does not undergo biological degradation.
3. The concentrations of most trace elements are relatively high in hair, as compared to the rest of the body.
4. Hair tissue provides a record of past as well as present trace element exposures.
5. Specimens of hair tissue can be collected more quickly and less invasively than specimens of other biological samples.

Pharmaceuticals, Contraceptives and Hair Minerals

It should also be pointed out that drugs and various pharmaceutical preparations can, in fact, also influence trace mineral levels. Recent work in our laboratory has indicated that patients who are on diuretics often have elevations in hair sodium or potassium levels. This indicates that influences of a pharmaceutical at the kidney level can have effects upon the transport and deposition of the alkaline metal family into the hair. Even in the face of relatively normal serum levels of sodium and potassium, one may still see greatly altered levels of sodium and potassium in hair mineral specimens. This would indicate that in the case of the alkaline metal families the hair may serve as an excretory route and be an early warning sign of alkaline metal wasting.

Deeming and Weber[23] have recently found that oral contraceptives also change the levels of trace elements in hair. Examination of Figure 9 shows that women taking oral contraceptives versus non-pregnant controls have higher zinc levels and lower hair copper levels, whereas their serum levels are exactly reversed with the non-pregnant controls having higher serum zincs and lower serum coppers.

Again, this reflects the interesting inverse relationship between serum levels of a trace element and hair levels of that same element in question. If, in fact, hair copper levels are reflective of liver copper levels, then this may suggest that women taking oral contraceptives have greater copper wasting from the liver and reduced microsomal enzyme function. The work of Cartwright and Wintrobe and Wintrobe et al in adult females has suggested that serum copper levels are proportional to circulating oestrogen levels.[24,25,26]

The results of Deeming and Weber, therefore, would indicate that as the serum levels of copper increase the liver may become depleted of copper and the hair levels subsequently indicate this loss by showing reduced levels as well. It is interesting to also note in Figure 9 that the dietary copper intake of the oral-contraceptive users was lower than the control women, suggesting that there may be more opportunity for depletion in that the copper is being utilized more rapidly in the oral-contraceptive-taking women, yet the dietary intake is less than 1.4mg/day, which suggests that

EFFECT OF ORAL CONTRACEPTIVES ON MINERAL LEVELS

Subjects	No. of subjects	Hair				Serum				Dietary			
		Fe	Mg	Cu	Zn	Fe	Mg	Cu	Zn	Fe	Mg	Cu	Zn
		ppm				μg/100 ml				mg/day			
Non-pregnant control women	7	62^{α}	54^{α}	70	199^{α}	106^{α}	1908^{α}	203	186^{β}	17^{α}	247^{α}	2.0^{α}	10^{α}
Women taking oral contraceptives	7	73^{α}	70^{α}	34^{α}	233^{β}	109^{α}	1813^{α}	348^{β}	149^{α}	36^{α}	230^{α}	1.4^{α}	11^{α}
SEM		16	7.8	18	7.3	11	44	9.3	6.5	13	35	0.19	1.4

$^{\alpha,\beta}$ Means having different superscripts are significantly different at the 0.05 level of probability.

Figure 9

depletion may occur upon long-term therapy of this type.

It also has been found that the use of one element in therapy may alter another element in question, showing both clinical manifestations of depression and reflection in the hair trace element patterns. An example of this is the report by Porter and Hemes et al[27] concerning the patient who presented herself with profound hypochromic macrocytic anaemia and associated cardiac failure. She had been on a long-term oral programme of zinc supplementation (660mg daily as the sulphate heptahydrate) for non-responsive coeliac disease. Upon examination of this patient it was found that her haemoglobin was 5.2g/dl, white cells 1.9 million, hematocrit of 0.21, and a mean cell volume of 109. Her serum zinc was 84mcg per 100ml and serum copper 40mcg/ml(normal 80 to 140). The hair copper was found to be .98mg per cent (normal 1.4 to 2.6).

It was therefore the suggestion that the large amount of zinc which she was ingesting for treatment of the coeliac disease was depressing her serum copper and reflected in her hair copper levels being very low. The therapy of choice was to remove her from the zinc supplements and give her 5mg of copper per day. Within three months her haematological picture had returned to normal and her hair levels had also returned to normal. Once again it illustrates the usefulness of hair trace mineral analyses in picking up apparent trace mineral metabolic patterns.

The Concern Over Analytical Procedures

The remaining problem which was mentioned by Lazar in his article, critical of hair tissue element analysis as a diagnostic tool, is that of the lack of standard analysis procedures and quality control standards within the commercial hair element testing laboratories. In the last year considerable progress has been made in standardizing the commercial hair washing, sample digestion, and analysis procedures for commercial hair element testing. The use of a standard washing procedure using an organic solvent, followed by an aqueous wash, is now employed by laboratories under the provisions of the protocols developed by the Hair Analysis Standardization Board and the Association of Elemental Substance Testing Laboratories, two professional organizations comprised of membership from the body of commercial hair element testing laboratories. The analysis procedure recommended by these groups follows that suggested by the International Atomic Energy Agency,[28] and has been spelled out in some detail in a recent article discussing the standardization of commercial hair element testing.[29]

Homogeneous powdered human hair samples are now available for standardization of techniques and quality control assessment within the industry. This should allow for much better correlations from laboratory to laboratory, and both inter- and intra-laboratory variations should be minimized. Laboratories are now accumulating data as it relates to the effects that various hair sprays and shampoos or hair treatments may have upon hair element concentrations, and a number of investigators have reported the importance of this information in interpreting hair element data.[30]

Screening for excess body burden of the toxic elements such as lead, mercury, cadmium, and arsenic by hair testing is now receiving much more attention, due to the understanding of the chronic, low level effects excessive levels of these elements have upon human function.

Recent data indicate that among children from six months to five years of age there is prevalency of greater than four per cent of elevated blood lead levels, and the suggestion is that excessive exposure to lead in the background environment may be a major community health problem.[31]

Needleman and Cohen have related excessive lead exposure and accumulation to such conditions as learning disabilities and autism.[32,33]

Low-level cadmium exposure has been found to induce specific functional and biochemical changes in the cardiovascular tissue of animals, indicating that ingested or inhaled low levels of cadmium may contribute to essential hypertension in humans.[34]

Shapiro and co-workers have found that dentists exposed to low levels of mercury have an occupational risk of adverse neurophysiological and psychological functions.[35]

Lastly, a condition resembling amyotrophic lateral sclerosis, or Parkinsonism, has been associated with exposure to aluminum.[36] Hair element screening has been found applicable to the assessment of excess body burdens of each of these toxic elements. Yokel has recently found that hair aluminum is a reasonable biopsy technique for establishing excessive exposure to aluminium, which when coupled with the previous work done on lead, mercury, cadmium, and arsenic indicate that if for no other reason hair element testing may be justified as a screening tool to determine excessive background toxic mineral exposure.[37]

It is clear from the past decade of hair element research that the relationship between hair element concentrations and human health and disease is a complex process that has to do with exposure, absorption, and tissue distribution of the various essential and toxic elements, which ultimately are reflected in different patterns of the hair. Many of these patterns are now beginning to be better understood and are proving to be useful information in the screening of individuals who may be suffering from trace element-induced metabolic imbalances.

At this point in time, the use of hair element testing as a screening tool for establishing excessive toxic metal body burden or defining potential imbalances of the essential trace elements seems justified. Many of the original criticisms offered by Dr Lazar concerning the applicability of the hair element testing technique have been adequately answered by research that has occurred since the publication of his article.

The future for hair element testing in preventive and predictive medicine appears very rich, and the rate at which the technique becomes more widely accepted depends to a great extent on the education of practitioners as to its utility and on the impetus for health scientists to engage in future research concerning the relationship between hair element concentrations and tissue levels of specific elements.

2.

THE UNIQUENESS OF HAIR AS A TISSUE FOR MINERAL BIOPSY

Over the past fifteen years it has become very apparent in the medical sciences that trace minerals exert an important and controlling influence on physiological function in the human. The mineral elements include calcium, magnesium, phosphorus, sodium, potassium, iron, copper, manganese, chloride, iodide, zinc, chromium, selenium, cobalt, and possibly vanadium, lithium, nickel, molybdenum, and even possibly a small amount of arsenic and silicon.[1] It is also known that not only do the cations play an important role but also the anions, such as iodine, chlorine, and even fluoride are important in the total control of physiological function.

As indicated in Figure 10, many metabolic problems are

SYMPTOMS OF TRACE MINERAL DEFICIENCIES

Element	Signs of Deficiency
Chromium	Glucose intolerance, insulin insensitivity
Cobalt	Pernicious anaemia, methylmalonic aciduria
Copper	Anaemia, leukopenia, neutropenia, Menke's syndrome
Iodine	Thyroid insufficiency, thyroglobulin
Manganese	Fatty acid metabolism dysfunction Mucopolysaccharide insufficiency
Selenium	Glutathione peroxidase insufficiency Increased lipid peroxidation and cardiac and muscle abnormalities
Silicon	Increased tendency toward atherosclerosis connective tissue dysfunction
Zinc	Impaired wound healing, hypogonadism, night blindness, dermatological changes

Figure 10

now well recognized as they relate to deficiencies of one or more of these essential trace elements in the human. Coupled with the increasing sensitivity of medical practitioners to the need for promoting proper essential trace mineral nutrition, is the heightened sensitivity to the role that excessive exposure to some of the toxic minerals such as cadmium, mercury, and lead have on producing dysfunction.

Dr Clair Patterson at the California Institute of Technology has found that even in one of the most pristine areas of the United States, Yellowstone National Park, there is still considerable enrichment of lead in the plants and animals as a result of fallout from the atmospheric dispersal of lead from our use of lead in fuels including petrol and coal.[2]

Taken together, then, it is clear that the assessment of both the essential minerals and the toxic minerals for a particular individual can be extremely important in establishing his or her own metabolic competency. Unfortunately, the symptoms which are associated with the chronic lack of one of the essential minerals or excessive amount of the toxic minerals can often be difficult to recognize and are only obviated at very grave states of deficiency or excess. It has become the responsibility of medical scientists to find better methods of early diagnosis of trace mineral inadequacy or toxic mineral excesses.

The past 20 years have witnessed the development of a technique to assess mineral status by measuring the enrichment of these elements in human head hair.[3] Unfortunately, however, as was pointed out in Chapter 1, there are several potential criticisms to the use of hair mineral testing to establish mineral adequacy. These include:

1. The variation in hair trace mineral levels as a result of different hair colours and beauty treatments to which the hair may be subjected.

2. The change in trace mineral levels of the hair as it reflects different washing procedures.

3. The effect of environmental perturbants such as aerosols from automobile exhausts and constituents of hard water.

4. The absence of the relationship between the hair trace mineral level and a tissue level of that same mineral.

5. The variation in mineral level as it relates to the colour of the hair and the condition of the scalp from which the hair was taken.

6. Variations in the control of the analytical technique used to determine the levels of trace elements in the hair.

As was explored in Chapter 1, each of these particular concerns can be adequately dealt with on the basis of data which are now available from contemporary research. Hair colour variation appears to be a minor consideration. Most beauty or cosmetic treatments of the hair do not significantly alter the trace element levels other than cold waving and bleaching.[4]

Washing the hair is generally not a serious problem if the appropriate preliminary washing procedure is used at the laboratory where the ultimate analysis is done.

Recently, relationships have been developed between the level of an element in the hair and the level of that same element in an organ or tissue of specific origin in the host.[5]

From these data, it can be surmised that the status of hair mineral diagnosis has changed considerably within the past ten years and it is now time to look seriously at its potential merit as a diagnostic screening tool for assessing either essential trace mineral adequacy or excessive toxic mineral exposure.

The first question which need be answered is that of why look at hair and not blood or urine as an assessment for mineral status? As is well known with the situation of serum calcium or serum iron, the levels in the blood can many times not reflect the status of the individual in that the blood is heavily buffered against significant change in the concentration of a particular mineral. For instance, if there is a compromise in calcium status of the individual, rather than the serum level going down, calcium is localized from the skeletal reserve and the serum level remains constant.[6]

Secondly, the levels of minerals in the blood are generally very low (in the parts per million range or less) which makes the analytical problem of accurate analysis very difficult.

Head hair provides itself as a very suitable alternative to both blood and urine analysis by circumventing these problems. The hair is a stable tissue which is primarily made up of a specific protein called keratin, which is very high in the sulfhydryl amino acid cystine. This amino acid is able to provide itself as a fairly strong chelator (derived from the Greek word *chelus*, meaning claw-like), which can bind heavy metals in an ionic state very effectively in this protein. As a result of this unique composition of the hair protein, the level of minerals in the hair is between ten to fifty times higher than the level of that same mineral in blood or urine, thereby making the analytical procedure much more simple.

Thirdly, whereby the blood is buffered against change of a particular element, as it relates to change of the status of the host, the hair is exquisitely sensitive to changes in status of a particular element as it relates to the host. Work done by Dr Bryan Pate at Simon Fraser University has indicated that the level of minerals in hair can show changes in an hourly fashion which are indicative of the status of the growing hair protein shaft.[7] Hair is also biologically stable and can be stored for long periods of time for re-analysis. It is also very readily procured by a non-invasive technique at the nape of the neck, whereby blood analysis necessitates vena puncture and transportation of a biologically active material.

How the Hair Traps Minerals

In order to understand something about the status of minerals in human hair, it is important to know something about the structure of hair and how the hair protein is synthesized and traps minerals as it grows. The growth of some hair is hormone-dependent, such as pubic and axillary hair, beard and moustache hair, whereas the eyelashes, eyebrows, and, to a degree, head hair appear to be less dependent upon hormone output. The human scalp has approximately 100,000 hairs, slightly more for blondes and less for redheads, and about eleven per cent, or approximately 10,000, of these hairs are in a resting phase, contributing to an average daily hair loss by shedding of 100 hairs. The active hair is growing at an average rate of about .4mm to .5mm per day, so that within a month about one-half inch of new growth would appear. The growing hair follicle is richly supplied with blood vessels, and the blood which bathes the follicles contains an array of essential and potentially toxic trace minerals which are laid into the new growing hair protein as a function of the rate of growth of the hair and its sulfhydryl content.

Hormonal or other chemical influences on the follicle also influence the uptake of specific elements and lastly, the level of the element in question within the blood relates to the amount deposited in hair. It is well known that the rate of hair growth is influenced by such factors as age, race, sex, season of the year, nutrition, and hormonal status of the host. It is known that the energy of the metabolism of the hair follicle is to a great extent provided by glucose in the blood, and therefore alterations in blood glucose levels can alter the metabolism of the energy cycle of the hair follicle. A state of adrenal insufficiency is known to be accompanied by a reduction of the amount of pubic and axillary hair, and this may be related to both the direct hormone involvement and the effects the glucocorticoids have upon glucose metabolism.

Because hair is almost predominately protein, changes in the protein nutritive status of the host can alter the composition of the hair and its growth rate and therefore influence the trace elements deposited in the hair. Changes in hair structure that are known to be associated with protein malnutrition include changes in the hair diameter, the growth rate, and differences in its tensile strength. Crounse and Van Scott have shown that the hair root protein is a more sensitive indicator of protein metabolism and malnutrition than serum albumin or transferrin.[8] Hair is composed of epithelial cells arranged in three layers: the cuticle, the cortex, and the medulla. The cortex forms the main bulk of the hair. It is a column of epithelial cells that is formed into a rigid homogenous mass. In the newly emergent hair the cortex has irregular shaped cells which carry tissue fluid.

As the hair continues to grow, the hair shaft dries out and the cavities lose their fluid, presumably losing fluid transport properties. The chemical structure of this protein material in the cortex, called keratin, is very similar to the protein of dental enamel and fingernails. It has been found that when you take human hair and treat it with the cold waving lotions or hair bleaching solutions, some synthetic organic hair dyes or depilatories, a marked depletion of cystine (one of the sulphur-containing amino acids) is observed. This changes the physical characteristics of the hair and markedly alters its ability to bind trace elements. This is one of the major reasons why hair taken from individuals who have bleached or cold waved their hair should be looked at with caution as it relates to trace mineral diagnostic usefulness.

The pigment in the hair is believed to be produced in cells of the hair bulb and continues to be formed in the cells of the cortex. This pigment is a relative of the skin pigment melanin, which is derived by way of a series of metabolic steps from the essential amino acid tyrosine through the action of a specific enzyme called tyrosinase. The greying process of hair is supposedly the result of a gradual loss of the tyrosinase activity over time, with the consequent inability to make hair pigment. It has been found that the pigment in red hair — called trichosiverin — is an iron-containing pigment. This may be one of the reasons that red-haired individuals often have slightly higher levels of iron than brown- or blonde-haired individuals.

Mineral Elements Deposited in the Hair

The mineral elements deposited in hair during protein synthesis have been studied for some time.[9] Early researchers have established water and ash content in hair, as well as aluminum, arsenic, bromine, calcium, chlorine, cobalt, copper, iron, manganese, nickel, phosphorus, lead, sulphur, uranium, and zinc contents. At the present time, some 27 elements have been identified in human hair in concentrations ranging from 0.1 to 100 micrograms per gram (ppm). The great majority of these trace elements in human metabolism serve chiefly as key components of enzyme systems, entitled metalo-enzymes. These minerals serve as facilitators for these enzymes, and in their absence the enzymes are either unable, or have a reduced ability, to perform their required function. It is well established now that metalo-enzymes have this function in the tissues.

Does a deficiency or an excess of one of these minerals in the hair of an individual indicate an alteration of a specific metalo-enzyme function within the tissues? The objective of the research workers in the field of hair trace mineral analysis in the past several years has been to attempt to identify the relationship between a specific mineral in the hair and a specific metalo-enzyme in a peripheral tissue. For some time it was felt in the hair trace mineral field that if an element was found in a higher than normal level in the hair, the individual must have had a margin of safety in regard to the reserve of that element, and there was no concern about the status of that specific element. However, as has been shown by Dr Jacob recently, this is truly a naïve position, in that high levels of elements, such as zinc, can often be as indicative of tissue deficiencies of that specific element as can low element levels.

A case in point to demonstrate this was that reported by Jacob and his co-workers of a 16-year- old young man who had suffered a traumatic head injury, had been comatose for some time, and had developed a decubitus ulcer and eczema. He showed very high levels of zinc in his hair — about 320 ppm (normal range, 160-240). He was given an oral zinc supplement, and over a period of the next six weeks his hair trace mineral level of zinc fell on a weekly basis. The week after the initial oral administration of zinc, his hair zinc rose from 320 to 390 ppm and then, following the same oral enrichment of zinc, the level of zinc in the hair ultimately returned back to a normal range of 180 ppm where it stayed. During the same period of time on therapy his decubitus ulcer cleared, as did his eczema. A phytohemmaglutinin challenge test was performed before and after therapy to measure his immune competence, recognizing that zinc is an extremely important element for stimulating immune systems, and it was found that whereas his immune competency was very low pre-therapy, after therapy his competency was that of the control.[10] This was a clear indication that high levels of a specific trace element in hair can be as indicative of a tissue mineral imbalance as low levels.

Hair tissue mineral analysis is a measurement of the intracellular level of a particular element, and therefore high levels may indicate a disproportionate deposition intracellularly of a mineral in a specific tissue, which then may cause a deficiency of that element in another tissue. The important question, then, is one of balance, as it relates to any specific element, and the maintenance of a relationship to other elements within a normal reference range. Work which has gone on during the past five years indicates the strong possibility that trace element content of hair correlates with body stores of specific elements, that the analysis of faeces and urine are of limited value as indicators of stores, and that blood is of restrictive use because the homeostatic mechanisms operate to keep the components of blood constant.[11]

Human head hair is a recording filament that reflects metabolic changes of the elements over a long period of time; therefore, it is a record of past nutritional events. Dr Gordus at the University of Michigan has examined the hair trace mineral content of naval midshipmen and West Point cadets and has tried to establish an optimal range for each of the selective elements, based upon this population group. It is interesting to note that when the incoming cadets first arrive at the academies, they have widely different trace element contents of their hair, presumably reflecting the difference in their past environmental and nutritional exposures. As they remain at the academies, however, their hair trace mineral patterns become more and more similar, demonstrating clearly that the environment, not the genetics of the individual, is one of the major controlling parameters, as it relates to trace element content of the hair.

It should be recalled, however, that the level of elements in the hair is not solely related to the nutritional status of that particular element in question. Dr Stanley Gershoff and his co- workers have found, for instance, that when they take rats and feed them diets all with the same level of trace elements, but with different amounts of protein, carbohydrate, fat, or vitamins, they can alter the level of elements in the hair considerably.[12] This suggests that it is not just the level of elements in the diet that controls hair mineral level, but rather the subjects' absorptive ability and their deposition of minerals in the hair follicles, as it relates to the total complement of other nutrients, including fat, protein, carbohydrate and the vitamins.

Hair element profiles should not be looked at as the sole screening device for assessing the mineral status of the diet. They are rather indicators of general metabolic activity of the individual, relating to the intra/extracellular partitioning of elements. It is also known that the mineral pollution of the environment contributes to the body burden of specific elements and can alter hair element levels.[13]

Toxic elements in the environment, such as lead, can result in human exposure, leading to an increase of those elements in the hair. There are two mechanisms by which these elements may arrive in the hair. One is by ingestion or inhalation, whereby the level of that element actually is found in the hair as a result of deposition through systemic processes, and the second is that of absorption of the toxic element from fallout onto the surface of the hair.

These two mechanisms of enrichment of the hair can be termed 'endogenous' and 'exogenous'. Endogenous refers to the fact that the element has to come into the body and arrive in the bloodstream before it could be deposited in the hair, whereas exogenous refers to the absorption onto the surface of the hair.

In most cases, the hair mineral pattern is used as a tool to assess systemic levels of a particular element, and therefore the exogenous forms of the element which are bound to the surface of the hair are of less importance than are the endogenous levels, which reflect body stores or burden. To separate the endogenous from the exogenous contributors, the hair is washed after arriving at the commercial testing laboratories, thereby freeing it of the absorbed form of the element and leaving primarily the endogenous element residue.

There are several different washing procedures that can be utilized, each with different effects upon different elements, due to different partition coefficients between the endogenous and exogenous forms in different solvents. In general, an aqueous wash of some type utilizing a detergent-type material seems to be an effective way of removing the exogenous absorbed forms of the elements, while leaving the systemically deposited endogenous forms.[14]

It has been found that the level of trace elements along hair from the scalp to the distal tip are not constant, but vary. Generally speaking, the portion of the hair which is most useful for assessing the systemic status of a particular element is the newest hair growth, which is the first inch to inch-and-a-half of growth from the scalp. As the hair gets longer, it has more opportunity to undergo environmental permutations which alter the level of elements in the hair. It should be stressed that, for accurate reproducible results of hair mineral patterns, the hair should be taken with the first inch or inch-and-a half of growth cut off and saved, and the remainder of the hair discarded. The analysis should then be done on this short section closest to the scalp.

Due to the fact that trace elements in hair are influenced by the metabolic status of the individual, it should also be recalled that pharmaceutical medications can also alter the level of trace elements in hair. The work of Drs Weber and Deeming have shown that very significant changes in zinc, copper, magnesium and iron content of the hair are found in women who have been treated with oestrogen — contained in oral contraceptives.[15] This is to be expected, in that hair growth is at least partially responsive to oestrogenic hormones, as well as general partitioning of minerals in various tissues.

As Thomas Maugh tells us in a recent article published in *Science* magazine and titled: 'Hair: A Diagnostic Tool that Complements Blood, Serum and Urine', hair mineral testing is a convenient, reasonably inexpensive, reproducible technique that can be utilized for assessing various aspects of mineral status of a patient, but is not in itself a panacea which allows complete understanding of the metabolic competency of the patient.[16] When used, however, in conjunction with blood, serum, urine, and dietary data, it provides itself as a powerful diagnostic modality which gives available information to the practitioner and which would not be easily procured by any other current technique.

Questions which must be explored to fully appreciate the impact of this technique include the problems of reproducibility and precision, recognition of diagnostic significance of hair mineral patterns and their relationship to specific disease states, and integration of these values with serum, urine, and dietary data to help in differential diagnosis and patient management.

These questions will frame the direction for the next Chapter. In summary, it can be said at this point that hair is a unique tissue for trace mineral biopsy, and its application to the medical sciences will continue in the future as we learn more about the power which it holds.

3.
HAIR MINERALS AS A SCREENING TOOL FOR TOXIC MINERAL EXPOSURE

Hair has the remarkable potential to become a useful diagnostic tool in clinical medicine. It is easily collected without trauma on the part of the donor, it can be stored without deterioration, and its contents can be analyzed relatively easily. Much of the original interest in hair mineral analysis surrounded the potential use of hair minerals as a screen for exposure of an individual to toxic minerals such as lead, mercury, cadmium, arsenic, and selenium. It is well known that Napoleon's hair, which was analyzed in 1961, contained at least 100 times the usual value for arsenic that would be considered normal, and it is suspected that he may have been killed by arsenical poisoning over a period of time, and that would explain his poor digestion and the necessity for his hand being placed over his abdomen frequently.[1]

More recently Kopito et al, at the Massachusetts Institute of Technology have suggested that hair mineral analyses may be the simplest and surest way to detect occult lead toxicity.[2] Positive results in screening for heavy metal toxicity have been obtained with elements such as lead, arsenic, cadmium, and mercury. Several investigators in Japan, Sweden, Canada, and the United States have shown that concentrations of these elements in the hair provide an accurate and relatively permanent record of exposure, and that there is a good correlation between concentrations in hair and specific concentrations in various organs.

The work of Dr Amares Chattopadhyay, who found that the concentration of lead in hair was lowest in rural population groups, higher in urban groups, and highest in individuals who live close to lead smelters, provides an example of the usefulness of the hair mineral screening technique. In his work he also observed the highest concentrations of mercury and cadmium in hair to be

COMMON SOURCES OF TOXIC MINERALS

Aluminium	Cookware Antacids Antiperspirants Aluminium cans
Arsenic	Insecticides Wine Well water Coal burning Seafood (particularly shellfish)
Cadmium	Water from galvanized pipes Evaporated milk Shellfish Cigarette smoke Sewage sludges Paint pigments
Copper	Copper plumbing Sewage sludge Beer Swimmming pools Copper cookware Mineral supplements
Lead	Atmospheric exhaust Paint Plumbing Tuna fish (canned) Hair dyes (lead acetate) Newsprint Lead shot Canned juice or fruit
Mercury	Dental fillings Seafood from bottom of ocean Treated seed grain Polluted water Skin lightening creams Sewage sludge

Figure 11

associated with individuals with known exposure to these elements.[3] Figure 11 lists the most common origins of exposure in the environment to most of the toxic minerals in human hair. High arsenic levels in the hair of residents of Yellow Knife, in Canada's Northwest Territory, and increased levels of arsenic, antimony, and cadmium in the hair were attributed to refinery emissions in the Toronto area.[4,5]

Recently, extensive work has been done on generalized community background lead excessive exposure and chronic toxicity, particularly in children. The exposure to lead, both in the working place environment and in the community background air and water as well as food, has led to the potential recognition of lead toxicity as a national health problem. The difficulty has been in establishing a proper screening test which can be utilized for selecting those people who may be subject to chronic lead-induced neurological or physiological impairment.

Many laboratory tests have been recommended for monitoring factory workers exposed to lead. In a recent study by researchers at the National Research Institute for occupational diseases in South Africa, 639 lead-exposed workers in several factories were questioned concerning the classic symptoms of lead intoxication, including abdominal aches, constipation, and fatigue, and were examined for hand tremor. Laboratory tests such as packed cell volume, blood lead, urinary lead, and delta-aminolevulenic acid were estimated in 489 workers. About half of the values for the blood tests fall into the excessive or dangerous category for lead absorption; however, no single test or group of tests was able to properly differentiate and pick up those people suffering from chronic lead exposure. Blood lead was found to be a better predictor of actual lead-induced symptomatic illness than any other laboratory test; however, it did not add appreciably to the prediction of potential illness. The suggestion from this work is that the effect of lead on illness does not appear to depend upon its action on the synthesis of red blood cells, and therefore basophylic stippling may not be requisite for diagnosing lead toxicity.[6]

A better assessment tool for chronic lead exposure would therefore seem to be that of hair mineral lead levels. Generally, hair mineral levels of lead in excess of 5mg per cent, or 50 parts per million, would be considered in the suspect area, and therefore those patients should be committed to additional testing to confirm the presence of lead toxicity. These should include haematological tests and specific enzyme tests, as well as blood lead levels. Because of the ambiguity in potential hair lead contamination as the result of the absorption of lead to the surface of the hair from some hair creams, an elevated hair lead should be confirmed by a pubic hair lead determination to guard against the possibility of hair preparation contamination of the sample.

Today world lead production is about 2.5 million tons per year, with approximately 40 per cent being used in the United States. Since 1940, there has been a marked increase in the production of lead as a petrol additive, which contributes to approximately 98 per cent of the airbourne lead.[7]

Recent work indicates that the level of biologic lead in the bones of present-day people is approximately a thousand times higher today than it was 1,600 years ago, suggesting increased accumulation of lead in our society in the biological food chain and potential increased toxicity as a result.[8]

A major form of studies published to date has been the use of blood lead concentration, often as a single value, as an index of previous exposure to lead. Recent studies have indicated that blood lead is not a reliable index of past absorption or toxicity per se.[9]

Dr Clair Patterson at California Institute of Technology has recently found that much of the excess lead body burden in children may contribute to chronic lead toxicity and may come from lead-contaminated canned tuna, which exceeds the natural concentration of lead in the fresh tuna by some 10,000 fold.[10] The magnitude of this source of lead helps explain the difference between lead concentration in the diet of present-day Americans at .2 parts per million and that of prehistoric peoples, which has been estimated at less than .002 parts per million.

The lead contamination appears to come from the seams of the cans in which tuna is stored, in that the flux used for solder contains lead as a flow agent. Also, the lead in the 'first flush' water coming from lead hot water pipes is much higher in lead than water taken after the faucet is run for a while. Consuming water that would be taken from a first flush water sample would provide much greater body burden of lead than would water taken from the same tap that had been running for some time.[11]

The impact of these major sources of lead background exposure on children seems to be centred on behavioural and psychological dysfunction. Several recent reports have indicated the relationship between lead exposure of a chronic nature and mental dysfunctional effects on children.[12,13,14]

Dr Herbert Needleman and his co-workers at the Mental Retardation Research Unit at the Children's Hospital in Boston have studied the relationship between lead accumulation in children in the dentine of their deciduous teeth and their performance on a standardized intelligence scale. It was concluded from this study that lead exposure at doses below those producing classic symptoms severe enough to be diagnosed clinically as lead toxicity appear to be associated with neuropsychological deficiencies that may interfere with classroom performance by preventing the child from being able to stay at task for an extended period of time by impairing concentration.

As the level of lead increased in the dentine of the teeth, the impairment increased, but of the students examined only two of them had what would be considered classic signs of lead toxicity.[14] This observation was further confirmed by the work of Doctors Pihl and Parkes at McGill University in Canada, who found that learning disabled children had much higher hair lead than did control children, who scored better on standard intelligence tests. These studies do not unequivocally demonstrate causality between learning impairment and lead increases, but do strongly suggest that lead may play a role in neurologic impairment and can be screened for easily by hair mineral testing.[15]

Lastly, it should be pointed out that lead is found in certain hair preparations up to concentrations as high as 3 per cent. It has been found that not only do hair preparations contain lead, but also certain cosmetics contain lead and can contribute to lead accumulation.[16] Some of this lead has been found to be absorbed across the scalp and can contribute to elevated blood lead levels. Therefore, elimination of lead-containing hair preparations can reduce systemic lead body burden.[17]

In the incidence of cancer in people who have been chronically exposed to background lead, both lead smelter workers and battery plant workers have been found to have increased cancer death rates, so screening by hair mineral testing could be very important in picking up occupational risks in these population groups to carcinogenesis induced by lead.[18]

Mercury Toxicity

Of the same degree of major concern as it relates to toxicity is mercury. One occupational risk group to mercury toxicity is made up of dental hygienists and chairside assistants, who are known to be exposed to higher amounts of mercury as the result of working with amalgams. It has been found that the most toxic part of the mercury exposure is not the inorganic mercury itself, but rather the conversion in the body to organic mercury forms such as methylmercury, which is the compound intimated to be involved with the Minimata disease in Japan.

In a recent study in which methylmercury levels were looked at in the blood of dentists, it was found that their total mercury levels were almost double that of their patient controls, but their methylmercury levels were fivefold higher than those of patient controls (dentists 24.7 ng/g vs. controls 4.7 ng/g).[19] These observations suggest that chronic mercurialism in dentists and others exposed to mercury vapour may be attributed to the effects of methylmercury and may be potentially screened by using hair tissue mineral analysis. Many of the symptoms of chronic poisoning by mercury, including depression, irritability, failure of memory and concentration, and hand tremor are also found in victims of methylmercury poisoning. Methylmercury, which is a fat-soluble substance has a particular affinity for brain tissue and can have influences on the central nervous system at low levels which cannot be seen easily through discreet symptomatology.

Cadmium

Cadmium has also been found to be an increasing problem as it relates to toxic mineral exposure. Combustion of coal and oil contributes to levels of cadmium in the environment, with the major amounts to which people are exposed today found in tobacco and canned foods. Both lung and kidney dysfunction have been observed in people suffering from cadmium exposure. Autopsy studies have revealed increased cadmium levels in individuals who have had emphysema, hypertension, and musculo-skeletal disease. The total body burden of cadmium is increased considerably by cigarette smoking and is found to be 19.3mg for non-smokers and 35.5mg for smokers. [20] Cigarette smoking results in the absorption of approximately 1.9mcg of cadmium per pack, as compared to dietary absorptions on the average of 2.7mcg per day. The half time for cadmium in the body is on the average 15.7 years; therefore, once accumulated it can have a long-term effect on physiology.

Aluminium

Another toxic element which may be screened effectively through the use of hair mineral levels is that of aluminium. Aluminium has traditionally been considered inert and therefore is now found ubiquitous within the environment, as a result of that supposition. As the result of the recent observations of aluminium fume fever and aluminium-induced dialysis dementia, aluminium has recently come under attack as a potential toxic element in the environment.[21] Excess aluminium concentrations which would be greater than 50 parts per million, or 5mg per cent, in the hair may be associated with excess body burden of aluminium, which increases parathyroid hormone output and may encourage osteolytic changes of bone with decalcification of hard tissue.[22] Recent work by Dr Kwang-Ming Chin, acting officer in charge of the National Institute of Neurological Disease and Stroke Research Centre in Guam, has found that cases of what appear to be amyotrophic lateral sclerosis in Guam residents may, in fact, be the result of aluminium-induced toxicity.[23] Alzheimer's disease-like symptoms with memory loss and neurologic impairment seemed to result from accumulated aluminium exposure. Although work needs to be done to unequivocally confirm that hair mineral testing is an appropriate screening tool for aluminium excess body burden, the preliminary evidence does seem to suggest the usefulness for hair mineral testing as a general screening tool.

Copper and Selenium

Two additional potentially toxic elements which merit mention are copper and selenium. A conspectus of the research on copper metabolism by Dr Karl Mason indicates that there are many neurological impairments associated with copper toxicity, not the least of which are the classic signs of Wilson's Disease. Copper metabolic problems have traditionally been assessed by the use of the enzyme ceruloplasmin, which is the major extracellular binding site of copper. It is well known that people with depressed ceruloplasmin levels may have accumulation of copper in their liver and neurological tissue which can cause cirrhosis-producing metabolites with neurological impairment.[24] Levels of copper in the hair in excess of 50 parts per million, or 5mg per cent, have been associated with suggestive excess body burden of copper. Behaviour changes and personality aggressiveness seem associated with these excess levels of copper. Again, hair mineral testing has been suggested as a reasonable screen for the status of body burden and specifically hepatic copper stores.[25]

Selenium is also an element which can become potentially toxic in excess levels. The provisional Recommended Dietary Allowance for selenium is approximately 120mcg per day. Levels above this can cause gastro-intestinal disturbances, neurological impairment, eyesight changes, and dermatitis.

Certain anti-dandruff preparations contain selenium and this can be, in sensitive individuals, an irritant, which may encourage dermatitis rather than successfully treat the dandruff, due to selenium sensitivity. In people utilizing selenium-containing hair preparations the level of selenium in the hair has little relationship to systemic levels of selenium and therefore should be viewed with caution. A recent report has indicated that selenium deficiencies may be picked up by low hair selenium levels, and the suggestion then is that possibly elevated hair selenium would be associated with selenium toxicity, although this remains to be confirmed.[26]

In conclusion, then, we can say that in screening for potential excess body burden of the toxic elements, including arsenic, lead, cadmium, mercury, aluminium, copper, and selenium, hair tissue mineral analysis may provide the most convenient, inexpensive, and readily available tool. By itself, it does not stand as a confirmation test for mineral toxicities, but rather is used as a first step in screening a patient for potential chronic exposure to excess toxic minerals. On the basis of this information alone, the expenditure of time, energy, and money on a hair mineral profile may be justified due to the ever-increasing prevalence of toxic mineral accumulation in our society.

4.

HAIR MINERAL PATTERNS AND THEIR RELATIONSHIP TO PHYSIOLOGY

The significant increase in appreciation of the role that trace elements play in human health and disease has led health practitioners to demand better ways of assessing mineral status in their patients.[1] Hair mineral testing provides itself as a potentially useful technique, in that hair is easy to obtain, store, transport, and relatively easy to analyse, thereby providing significant information about trace mineral status, both of the essential and the toxic mineral families.

A variety of the problems which have encumbered the development and acceptance of the hair mineral testing technique have been resolved within the past few years by extensive research.[2] The more common human nutritional essential elements, which include calcium, magnesium, sodium, potassium, iron, copper, chromium, manganese, zinc, and selenium, have all been found to have some relationship between their levels in hair and potential specific human pathological conditions. It has been well established that human head hair is an excellent biopsy tissue for the assessment of potential toxic mineral exposure as the result of environmental pollution.[3] Those individuals in Japan who were exposed to methylmercury poisoning as a result of the Minimata Bay disaster were found to have significantly higher levels of mercury in their hair than a control group.[4] Dentists and chairside assistants have been found to be exposed to mercury background in the office as the result of amalgam utilization. It has been established that hair mineral testing is a reasonably good way of assessing the degree of mercury exposure and body burden in these dental personnel.[5] The effects of excess body burden of many of these toxic elements is initially that of neurological and psychomotor dysfunction, particularly in children who seem to have a greater sensitivity to excess toxic mineral exposure.

A house-to-house survey of children living in a rundown neighbourhood of Boston noted 23 to 27 per cent of the children having minor neurologic dysfunctions and motor impairment. The evaluation of the lead status of these children indicated that they had increased lead body burden and upon treatment to remove the lead from their systems certain measurements of intellectual performance were enhanced.[6]

Recently, Needleman and co-workers, in a study done in the Boston metropolitan area, found that elevated lead in the dentine of the teeth of school children was correlated with impairment in learning and behaviour. Of the 2,146 children studied, only two have frank plumbism, as measured by enzyme tests, or basophilic stippling of their red blood cells. The remainder of the children had differing degrees of chronic lead intoxication, which resulted in differing degrees of neurologic impairment, which was first seen as the child's inability to stay at a task, or concentrate. A child at school who cannot concentrate for any prolonged period is often labelled by the teacher as being hyperactive or learning-disabled, and, as a result, is selected out of the normal classroom situation for special programmes. The conclusion drawn from Needleman's work is that there is a potentially significant problem in the U.S.A. with regard to lead intoxication of a chronic nature in American youngsters.[7]

This conclusion is further confirmed by the work of Drs Pihl and Parkes at the Psychology Department of McGill University. In their studies they took hair samples from 31 learning- disabled children and 22 normal children who were sex-, age-, socio-economically-, and language- matched and determined the content of 14 elements within the hair. Significant group differences were found at the .001 confidence level, with one of the more important differences being a much higher lead level (approximately four times higher) in the learning-disabled group versus the control group of children. Utilizing these differences in trace elements within the hair, these workers were able to separate children who would be learning-disabled or control children upon testing, on the basis of their hair mineral patterns alone.[8]

Lewis Kopito and his co-workers have confirmed the

importance of hair as a screening tool for lead toxicity. They conclude that the determination of lead in scalp hair is a valuable diagnostic aid in chronic or mild lead intoxication, particularly when the other clinical or laboratory evidence is of questionable conclusions.[9] Because hair is a continuously growing tissue that accumulates lead for long periods and is useful, then for estimating the time and duration of the exposure. Similar conclusions have been drawn with regard to the elements cadmium, mercury, and arsenic.[10]

The question which commonly arises in the minds of clinicians as it relates to the usefulness of hair tissue mineral analysis data is that concerning the importance of relative ratios of one mineral to another in the hair. Creason and his co-workers have found that when you look at trace elements in hair the potentially most useful data come from utilizing relative ratios of elements one to the other, rather than just absolute values alone.[11]

CLINICALLY IMPORTANT HAIR MINERAL RATIOS

Ratio	**Ideal**	**Significance**
Zinc Copper	8:1	Cardiovascular, female reproductive system, liver function
Zinc Manganese	150:1	Musculo-skeletal, collagen, cholesterol biosynthesis
Zinc Calcium	3:1	Cardiovascular, osteodynamics, renal function
Sodium Potassium	2:1	Adrenal status, endocrine involvement
Calcium Magnesium	8:1	Cardiovascular, osteodynamics, dietary imbalance
Iron Copper	2.5:1	Haematological, energy production through respiration

Figure 12

Inter-element correlations indicate that the best element for ratio determination and normalization of values appears to be that of zinc. Therefore, zinc-to-copper, zinc-to-manganese, zinc-to-calcium ratios are of potentially significant diagnostic utility because they tend to balance out interlaboratory variations, and perturbations from environmental exposure, which may not be picked up by utilizing absolute values alone. Ideal reference ranges for ratios of various elements within hair are seen in Figure 12.

It may turn out that relative ratios are more indicative of trace element status of specific tissues in the human body than are whole blood serum or urinary trace mineral data, the latter having potentially small significance to specific clinical manifestations.[12] Hair mineral analysis has been found to be extremely useful in the establishment of several basic clinical manifestations of trace mineral imbalances. These include: Malabsorption syndrome, zinc-to-copper imbalances, endocrine problems, and excessive toxic mineral exposure.

Malabsorption

In certain clinical manifestations of malabsorption syndrome, such as cystic fibrosis in children it has been found that the hair patterns indicate significant alterations from normal reference values, both in terms of specific elements and ratios of elements. Lewis Kopito has found that the concentration of sodium, potassium, calcium, and magnesium in the scalp hair of neonates with cystic fibrosis are significantly elevated over control children, particularly that of sodium and potassium. Nearly all of the calcium and magnesium found in the hair of these children is extractable in boiling water, whereas only a small fraction of calcium and magnesium of the hair is extractable from healthy infants.

The inability of hair from patients with cystic fibrosis to bind calcium and magnesium may be related to the basic defect of the disease, alterations in protein synthesis of the hair. Therefore, low calcium, magnesium and elevated sodium/potassium in the hair is diagnostically useful for picking up cystic fibrotic conditions.[13]

Malabsorption of trace minerals can also occur as the result of hypochlorhydria, or poor stomach acid output.

Many of the polyvalent elements which have multiple oxidation states are absorbable in only one of their oxidation states, which is facilitated by lower pHs. Low stomach acid output, therefore, can render these elements less absorbable and the hair mineral profile will show this pattern as low values for these elements, such as iron, copper, manganese, chromium, and to a degree calcium and magnesium, which are not true polyvalent elements, but still seem to depend on acid for their absorption.

Patients who have significantly low levels of many of the heavy elements in their hair should be suspected of malabsorption syndrome, either as a result of poor stomach output, chronic pancreatic insufficiency, or gastro-intestinal mucosal changes which have prevented proper absorption. The latter syndrome often accompanies diets of high solute content, such as diets high in salt and sugar and low in fibre, which can flatten the gastro-intestinal villae and reduce the absorptive surface area.

Glucose Intolerances

Hair chromium has been found to be a useful indicator for potential glucose tolerance sufficiency within juvenile and maturity onset diabetics. Dr Michael Hambidge and his co-workers have reported that the concentration of chromium in the hair of juvenile-onset diabetics, as compared to control children, was found to contain much lower levels of chromium at a confidence limit of $P < .001$.[14] Little cause and effect have been unequivocally established between low chromium in the hair and chromium status being the cause of the diabetes; however, it has been found that the concentration of chromium in the hair of young women who have just given birth is significantly lower than mulliparous women of the same age group.[15] It has been suggested that the lower values in the parous group is a result of the depletion of tissue chromium stores during pregnancy in the potential formation of glucose tolerance factor in the liver of the foetus. If the mother is already compromised with regard to chromium, this may jeopardize the status of the neonate with regard to the accumulation of chromium in the last trimester of pregnancy and impair glucose tolerance.[16] This may be of even greater diagnostic significance when hair zinc is compromised. Diabetic children have been found to have much lower hair zinc concentrations before insulin therapy than either diabetics treated with insulin or healthy children (114 ppm versus 261 and 215 respectively).[17]

It would appear then that low hair zinc and low chromium are potentially diagnostically significant as it relates to glucose tolerance. This association between low levels of these elements in the hair and diabetes does not necessarily confirm causality, but it does raise very strongly the potential usefulness of the hair technique as a screening tool as well as opening doors for future research in the management of certain types of glucose intolerance which may be related to trace mineral insufficiencies.

Zinc and Copper Status

Zinc deficiency has been shown to be prevalent in soil, plants, and food and is probably widespread in humans in Western culture. Zinc deficiency syndromes include: poor wound healing, poor growth rates, taste imperception, slowing of hair growth rate, vitamin A non-responsive night blindness, dermatological problems, and increased risk of dental caries.[18]

Pioneering work by Dr William Strain found that hair tissue mineral analysis for zinc was simple, reliable, and non-traumatic measurement for assessing various aspects of body zinc status.[19] It has been found that levels of zinc in the hair less than 90 parts per million (9mg per cent) are suggestive of frank zinc deficiency in the adult human and have been found commonly in populations where there is prevalence of kwashiorkor. More recently, however, it has also been found that elevated hair zinc can also be associated with tissue zinc insufficiency. Therefore, levels above 260 ppm (26mg per cent) have also been found associated with tissue zinc insufficiency.[20] This apparent contradiction has been resolved by the fact that hair growth is intimately dependent upon zinc status, in that hair is a synthesized protein which depends upon zinc metalo-enzymes for its manufacture. Compromising the zinc status of an individual then leads to slower hair growth rate initially, which leaves the hair in longer residence time at the follicle with more opportunity to saturate with low levels of serum zinc and produces an elevated hair zinc level.

If the individual has been undergoing zinc deprivation for

a considerably longer period of time, however, the status of zinc may be so compromised that at that point the chronic deficiency of zinc may be reflected in an equilibrium exchange alteration which results in low hair zinc. The conclusion is that both elevated hair zinc and depressed hair zinc can be indicative of tissue zinc status insufficiency and can be approached by supplementation with zinc. These results help to resolve the conflicting information which has appeared in the literature recently which has shown no relationship between hair zinc levels and serum levels.[21,22]

As Dr Hambidge pointed out recently, low hair zinc and elevated hair zinc values which are reported in Hispanic American pre-school children of low height percentiles are more likely related to poor growth as a result of zinc deprivation than to genetic factors.[23] This would suggest strongly that hair zinc is an excellent screening tool for zinc status in youngsters who may be on zinc compromised diets, which result in an untoward effect either in growth or immune defence.

It should be noted that zinc and copper in the hair can also be altered by certain hair preparations. Two that have been found to have significant influence on hair zinc and copper status are bleaching, which reduces the level of both zinc and copper, and cold waving, which reduces zinc and elevates copper in the hair.[24] It should also be noted that the distance that the hair is taken from the scalp can have a significant influence on the level of copper and zinc in the hair. The best sample is the first inch and a half to two inches of growth from the scalp at the nape of the neck. Longer hairs have increased copper and zinc at the tips of the hair as a result of exogenous contamination and are not suitable for analysis.

It is also clear that water that is contaminated with copper, such as swimming pool water, can lead to synthetic elevations of hair copper. This has commonly been called the 'green hair syndrome' in swimmers.[25] The hair here has an extremely high affinity for copper and binds it very tightly even at low concentrations in the environment. Therefore, elevations of hair copper may be a result of cold waving, the use of long hair strands for analysis, or swimming pool exposure to copper. Once these sources of copper contamination have been eliminated, the hair tissue copper level can be a useful indicator of hepatic copper stores.[26]

Jacob and Klevay have suggested that the determination of copper in hair may be useful for assessing total liver copper content in humans and that the copper in the liver may participate in the control of plasma cholesterol through the conversion to bile acids and the ultimate excretion of cholesterol in that form. Figure 5 illustrates the inverse relationship between serum cholesterol and hair copper levels which seem to have confirmed this particular suggested correlation.

In a recent study by Epstein and co-workers, however, it was not found that humans who have cirrhotic liver condition, in which there is known copper accumulation in the liver, have elevated hair copper levels. In ten patients who had increased liver copper concentrations, only one had increased hair copper. Therefore, they come to the conclusion that in primary biliary cirrhosis hair copper does not reflect liver copper content and is of no value as a biopsy material for copper analysis.[27]

It has also been found that the copper content of hair in persons suffering from Wilson's Disease is not abnormal relative to control population, suggesting that certain kinds of liver pathology which are consistent with copper accumulation, may have different metabolic influences on hair copper from other manifestations of chronic alterations in proper copper metabolism[28] This position is advanced as a result of three additional observations. Deeming and Weber have shown that women taking oral contraceptives, which are known to reduce hepatic copper stores and increase serum cholesterol, have lower hair copper levels than do women not taking oral contraceptives.[29] It is interesting to note that women on oral contraceptives also have an increased risk of coronary heart disease which may suggest that hair copper levels may be a potential screening tool for oestrogen-induced increased risk to coronary heart disease.

It should be noted that pigmentation of the hair seems to have little influence on zinc and copper content. Recently, individuals who were found to have hypochromotrichia as a result of kwashiorkor, which is associated with a marked lightening of the hair colour to various shades of brown, red, blonde, or grey, did not have altered zinc or copper content of the hair, relative to the control population. [30]

The second observation which would confirm the fact that hair copper status is useful in assessing systemic copper status is the report that a woman who had been supplemented with large doses of zinc sulphate (220mg taken 3 times daily) had developed a hypochromic macrocytic anaemia and associated cardiac failure. It was found that she had a very depressed serum copper and depressed hair copper level and elevated serum zinc and hair zinc level. When the zinc supplement was removed and she was given copper, her haematological pattern cleared and her hair copper went from .9 to 2.3 ppm.[31]

Lastly, the third observation is of patients suffering from Menkes kinky hair syndrome, which is a progressive neurodegenerative disorder, associated with changes in copper status of the liver, were found to have very low copper levels in their hair.[32] Again, this would indicate that in chronic states of copper metabolic difficulties or dietary deficiencies the hair copper may be a useful tool for early recognition of the problem, whereas in cirrhotic liver conditions and Wilson's Disease hair copper may not be an adequate assessment tool.

The clinical manifestations of these observations may be that hair zinc and copper levels are a useful screening tool for potential cardiac irregularities or liver detoxification status. Dr Klevay has proposed that zinc and copper status is extremely important in establishment of a risk factor to coronary heart disease.[33] It has been shown that there is a direct relationship between the body's copper-zinc ratio and ventricular premature beats and a potential association of this with sudden coronary death.[34] This would suggest strongly that the hair zinc-to-copper ratio of 8 to 1 may be an extremely important benchmark in establishing proper mineral metabolism status for two trace minerals that are extremely important in both hepatic detoxification systems and clearance of serum cholesterol and other potential mutagenic agents from the liver.

The next chapter will trace other clinical uses of hair tissue mineral patterns in recognition of trace mineral-related degenerative diseases.

5.

INTEGRATION OF HAIR MINERAL DATA WITH SERUM, URINE AND DIETARY DATA

Examination of blood and urine provides immense insight into the presence of certain human diseases. In the early inception of the hair mineral analysis field it was natural to hope that the examination of human hair would also add to the power of these routine examinations in the diagnosis of disease. However, the problem is that analysis of the first inch to inch and a half of growth of the hair represents what has been happening metabolically to that patient over a three-month period, rather than at a single point in time, which is what the serum and urine provide. As a result of this, hair as a diagnostic tool is much more valuable as a general metabolic screening tool than as a discrete diagnostic criterion for disease.[1] Hair tissue mineral analysis data, together with urinary, serum, and dietary data, however, provide a powerful complementary system of modalities that allow the assessment of several features of the patient's unique physiologic process that can then be used for the construction or alteration of a more health-promoting lifestyle, as it relates to diet, exercise, stress reduction, and general life-style modification.

The philosophy underlying this preventive approach towards health care is that, by intervening in the basic metabolic deficiencies, an improvement in organ reserve can occur, throughout the years, which leads to enhanced ability to withstand physiologic stresses and to an increased ability to maintain homeostasis.[2]

The definition as to what represents an optimal level of the specific element in hair is constantly undergoing change as it relates to establishing a better optimum test reference population. There is a clear difference between the definition of a normal level in hair which represents the aggregate average of a specific element in an average population versus the optimal level which may be considered an ideal range that an individual should point toward. The definition of the normal level of an element in hair may be different for different geographical areas because of the strong environmental influences, whereas the ideal level of each specific element in human physiology would be a range that would account for biological variability but would represent levels suggestive of optimal physiological function for that person.

Because of differences in hair protein composition and genetic disorders of hair growth and also environmental permutations, it is reasonably clear that at this point hair does not represent a singular diagnostic modality which allows unequivocal assessment of physiological function, but is a complement to blood, urine, and dietary data in trying to paint a reasonable picture of where patients are as it relates to their biochemical uniquenesses and the responses of their physiology to their lifestyle. In managing a patient under this philosophy, therefore, it is important to collect not only hair tissue mineral data, but also a good medical and health history, a representative sample of blood and urinary analytic data, and lastly a dietary diary or diet record which would allow assessment of both the macronutrient and micronutrient inputs. The latter dietary evaluation is best accomplished by a computerized dietary survey which would be able to roughly quantify the intake of the various elements in the diet relative to one another and to the absolute recommended dietary allowance standards.

The importance of quantifying the environment of the patient is to be stressed in that a specific environment may contain agents or contaminants which alter physiological function and cause changes in the patient's dietary, serum, and hair data. A reasonable example of this is the fact that the mean lead levels of infants' head hair has been found to be higher in children whose mothers had high hair lead than in infants who were born of mothers with lower hair lead levels.[3] As the child aged and was removed from the mother's placental environment for some time, the hair lead level went down, suggesting that the elevated level was not the result of genetic tendencies toward higher concentration of lead, but rather to exposure during the foetal period from lead intake from the mother's diet or environment.

It is also interesting to note that the work of Dr Gordus on naval midshipmen and West Point cadets indicated that the longer they stayed at the academies the more similar their hair mineral levels became to one another, indicating that similar dietary and environmental histories are associated with similar types of mineral patterns.[4] The work of Gershoff et al in Thailand has also indicated that minerals in the hair are not directly correlated with dietary intake of that respective mineral but rather are related to the full complement of the diet and environment as it relates to the composition of protein, carbohydrate, fat, and vitamins, as well as the minerals in the diet.

In one series of studies done with rats, the Gershoff group could demonstrate a change in hair zinc concentration by a factor of two by altering not the zinc content of the diet, but rather by altering the protein and sugar concentrations of the diet. The high sugar diet led to low hair zinc whereas the higher-protein, lower-sugar diet led to higher hair zinc, even in the face of the two dietary regimes having virtually identical zinc content.

The key, then, is that the dietary survey can be utilized to assess the quality of the diet as it relates to not only the mineral composition but also as to the absorbability and utilizability of the minerals. This in conjunction with hair mineral data then allows assessment of the degree of mineral absorption and proper functional utilization of the respective minerals.

The power of the integrative diagnostic approach toward recognition of unique needs that a patient has with regard to his or her nutrition can be seen from a series of examples. One classic example is the patient who has a hair mineral zinc-to-copper ratio in excess of 12 to 1, with a hair zinc-to-manganese ratio in excess of 200 to 1, whose blood chemistry shows an elevation of serum cholesterol in excess of 210mg per cent and an elevated cholesterol to high density lipoprotein cholesterol ratio in excess of 5 (ideal is 3). This, in conjunction with symptoms of lower back pain and poor aerobic fitness, elevated blood pressure, and musculo-skeletal problems, can stongly suggest the need to assess the fats in the diet as well as the magnitude of manganese and zinc in the dietary intake. Elevated blood fats with reduced dietary fibre, in conjunction with decreased dietary manganese and zinc, contribute significantly to the kinds of patterns indicated in the previous example.

This patient is at greater risk to coronary heart disease problems and may have a mucopolysaccharide synthesis problem that leads to back and musculo-skeletal pain.

Utilizing a single piece of data, such as the hair, the diet survey, or the blood chemistry, would not have given the diagnostician the power that utilizing the three in conjunction, along with symptoms, does. This directs the clinician by redundancy of information toward a pertinent dietary management programme that is multi-factorial and allows for complementary components to be utilized in accentuating the patient's management. An addititional example would be the patient who has a reduced hair selenium with an elevated zinc-to-copper ratio in excess of 12 to 1 with symptomatic premature ventricular beats and shortened erythrocyte survival time which might be seen as a depressed red blood cell count and a tendency of the blood to hemolyze easily under oxidative stress. This type of pattern is classic in its association with reduced antioxidant defence systems that are mediated through vitamin E and glutathione peroxidase, which is a selenium-containing metalloenzyme.[6]

Work done in China has recently indicated that a type of cardiomyopathy in children, which has been entitled Keshan's Disease, is in part related to a selenium deficiency in the children's diet and which can be corrected by selenium supplementation.[7] This type of pattern may be a particular problem to a person who carries the genetic tendency towards glucose-6-phosphate dehydrogenase deficiency, which makes his or her blood already more susceptible to hemolytic oxidative damage.

Again, the importance of recognizing the marriage between genetics and the environment of a patient is important in establishing a risk factor for potential degenerative problems. This is the power of the health screening tool utilizing hair mineral analysis in conjunction with other accepted tests. The premature ventricular beats may well have been an early warning sign of copper deficiency.[8]

Considerable work done recently by Dr Leslie Klevay seems to suggest that copper deficiency may increase the risk of atherosclerosis and of particular types of cholesterolemic problems.[9]

Dr Klevay has suggested that hair mineral analysis may be

a useful technique for screening individuals for potential copper deficiency.[10] It should be pointed out, however, that there are two conflicting reports in the literature which have appeared recently, calling into question the ability of hair technique to establish copper status both in cases of cirrhosis, where the liver is known to accumulate copper, and in frank copper deficiency in a small number of neonates, where there was correlation between hair copper and body copper status.[11,12]

Once again, it would appear that hair is a more powerful technique for general screening than it is for the establishment of pathological states, as it relates to trace minerals. This is why the hair mineral ratios may prove more useful in establishing a pattern within the patient as it relates to intracellular levels and metabolic control of elements rather than singular levels of each of the elements.

Clinically Significant Patterns

In examination of the hair mineral data, there are four basic patterns which the clinician may find very useful at first inspection.

The first pattern has been discussed at some length in the previous articles, which is that of elevated toxic minerals, including lead, mercury, arsenic, cadmium, aluminium, and copper. Any one or more of these elements that are elevated into the suggested excessive range may be indicative of excessive mineral body burden. The signs and symptoms of each of these elements in the toxic range are as seen in Figure 13. The confirmation of an elevated level by pubic hair analysis and/or blood or urinary tests is very important before embarking on an aggressive treatment regime. Treatment generally employs the use of either oral or intravenous chelation agents, which help remove toxic minerals from the body. Oral chelation agents can be thought of as the sulphur-containing foods, rich in the amino acids cystine and methionine such as eggs, beans, onions, and garlic, as well as vitamin C-rich foods and the use potentially of antagonistic minerals such as calcium to displace lead, selenium to counteract mercury, and calcium/magnesium to counteract aluminium.

The second clinically useful hair pattern is that of low hair sodium, potassium, chromium, and manganese. This

TOXIC MINERAL SYMPTOMS

Mineral	Symptoms	Confirmatory Tests
Lead	tiredness, anaemia learning disabilities	Basophilic stippling of red blood cells, blood lead, blood protoporphyrin
Mercury	memory loss, hallucinations, peripheral neuropathy	blood mercury, pubic hair mercury
Cadmium	hypertension, kidney problems musculo-skeletal pain	urinary or blood cadmium pubic hair cadmium
Arsenic	anaemia, lassitude, easy fatigue, GI complaints	urinary arsenic after IV EDTA challenge
Copper	volatile personality, mood swings, schizophrenic type behaviour, speech difficulties	urinary copper after penicillamine challenge, pubic copper
Aluminium	memory loss,symptoms of presenile dementia, osteoporosis	no suitable alternative (tissue biopsy)

Figure 13

particular pattern is often correlated with the clinical manifestations of gulcose intolerance and significant deviation from an ideal six-hour oral glucose tolerance curve associated with this hair mineral pattern is that of a latent phase hypoglycemic rebound at the fourth or fifth hour of the test, which was preceded by a postprandial hyperglycemic rise, as seen in Figure 14. Using the hair mineral pattern of low sodium, potassium, manganese, and chromium, an individual then can be potentially screened for the need for an oral glucose tolerance type test to confirm this pattern of glucose intolerance. The dietary management can then be employed, using the higher complex carbohydrate, higher fibre dietary approach of Anderson.[13]

The third clinically useful pattern is that of an elevated hair calcium and magnesium level, with a calcium-magnesium ration in the deal range of 8 to 1. This type of pattern has been correlated [14] with condition of

RELATIONSHIP OF HAIR COPPER LEVELS
TO SERUM CHOLESTEROL

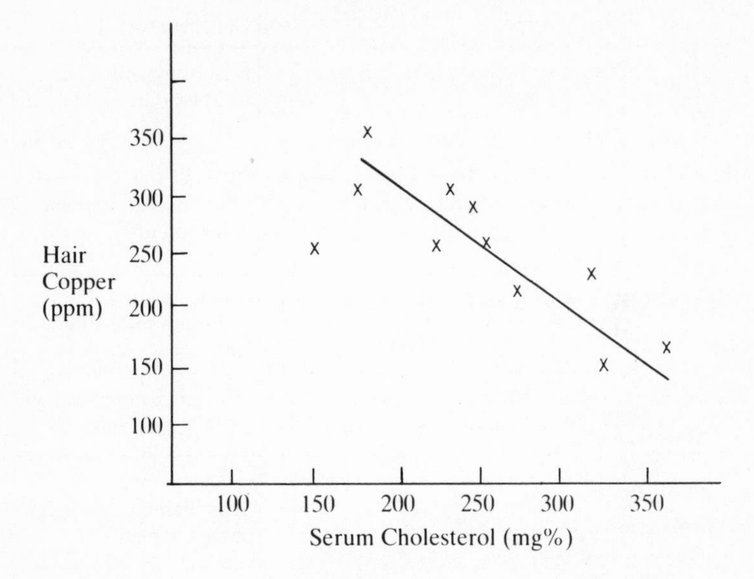

Figure 14

nutritionally-induced secondary hyperparathyroidism, with concommitant loss of calcium from bone stores. This may be a very important clinical profile, in that in many cases where an elevated calcium/magnesium hair level is seen, the blood serum shows calcium and phosphorus to be within normal range. However, this individual may, upon 24-hour urine studies of calcium spill, show altered urinary calcium output, indicating the borderline hyperparathyroid condition. The work done by Bland et al does, in fact, indicate that the reduced calcium-excessive phosphorus-rich diet, which many individuals are on, encourages the output of parathyroid hormone and the loss of calcium from bone stores, with concommitant increase in hair calcium and magnesium. The dietary management then is to use a higher alkaline ash diet with a calcium-phosphorus ratio of .7 to 1 or greater, rather than the average American calcium-phosphorus ratio of about .52 to 1.

The major difficulties with the average Western diet that account for the low calcium, excessive phosphorus in the diet are due to excessive red meat consumption, excessive processed foods which can contain phosphate additives, and lastly — and possibly most important — is the consumption of carbonated beverages, be they either sugar- or synthetically-sweetened. They all contain phosphorus as a buffering agent. Elimination, or at least control, of these particular dietary variables, as seen in the diet survey, with the addition of grains, vegetables, and cultured milk products will encourage the proper calcium-phosphorus dietary ratio and will improve calcium metabolism and status.

The fourth clinically important pattern from hair tissue mineral analysis is that of general low levels of many of the polyvalent elements, including copper, iron, manganese, chromium, and selenium. As these elements all become low in the hair pattern, it is often correlated with malabsorption syndrome, due to hypochlorhydria or other gastro-intestinally related malabsorption difficulties. The hypochlorhydria can be confirmed by nasogastric intubation, or by Heidelberg gastric acid secretion tests. In these patients the control of the diet, and even the use of very expensive supplements, may be in vain if the stomach acid sufficiency problem is not dealt with first. The status of the absorptive pathways will, to a great degree, determine the eventual nutritional outcome of that individual with respect to those specific items that are poorly absorbed. Confirmation of the malabsorption problem and dietary management thereof, using betaine hydrochloride or glutamic acid hydrochloride as acid replacement therapy, can be extremely important, particularly in the aged individual, in improving absorption and thereby improving nutritional status.

These four clinically relevant patterns are but a few of the types of screening tools available from the hair mineral profile. It should be noted, however, that none of those data should be used singularly, but rather in conjunction with blood, urinary, and dietary data, as well as clinical symptomatology. When put together, this programme frames a most useful diagnostic set of tools, which allow the clinician to assess and thereby manage specific nutritionally related problems of the patient which are not easily procured by other methodologies.

REFERENCES

Introduction

1. Gori, G. 'Macroeconomics of Disease Prevention', *Science*, 200 (1978), 1124.
2. Engel, G.L. 'The Need for a New Medical Model', *Science*, 196 (1977), 129.
3. Mertz, W. 'Trace Minerals', *Contemporary Nutrition*, 3 (1978).
4. Maugh, T. 'Hair: A Diagnostic Tool to Complement Blood, Serum and Urine', *Science*, 202, 1271-1274.
5. Klevay, L. 'Hair as a Biopsy Material. Progress and Prospects', *Arch. Intern. Med.,* 138 (1978), 1127-1128.

Chapter 1

1. Lazar, P. 'Hair Analysis: What Does it Tell Us?', *J. Am. Med. Assoc.,* 229 (1974), 1908.
2. Chittleborough, G. 'A Chemist's View of the Analysis of Human Hair for Trace Elements', *Science of the Total Environment*, 14 (1980), 53-75.
3. McKenzie, J. 'Alteration of Zinc and Copper Concentration of Hair', *Am. J. Clin. Nutr.,* 31 (1978), 470-476.
4. Kennington, G.S. 'Soluble and Fixed Elements in Mammalian Hair', *Science*, 155 (1967), 588-590.
5. Clegg, M.S., Keen, C.L. and Hurley, L.S. 'Influence of Washing Techniques on the Analysis of Trace Elements in Animal Tissue', *Biological Trace Element Res.,* 3 (1981), 107-115.
6. Maes, D. and Pate, B. 'Spatial Distribution of Copper in Individual Human Hairs', *J. Forensic Sci.,* 21 (1976), 127.
7. Jacob, R., Klevay, L. and Logan, G. 'Hair as a Biopsy Material: Index of Hepatic Copper', *Am. J. Clin. Nutr.,* 31 (1978), 477-481.
8. Pekarek, R.S., Sandstead, N. and Jacob, R. 'Abnormal Cellular Immune Response Acquired During Zinc Deficiency', *Am. J. Clin. Nutr.,* 32 (1979), 1466-1470.

9. Hambidge, K.M. and Rodgerson, D.O. 'Comparison of Hair Chromium Levels in Multiparous and Parous Women', *Am. J. Obstet. and Gynecol.,* 103 (1969), 320-324.
10. Gibson, R. 'Hair as a Biopsy Material for the Assessment of Trace Element Status in Infancy', *J. Human Nutrition,* 34 (1980), 405-416.
11. Bergmann, K.F., Makosch, G. and Tews, K.H. 'Abnormalities of Hair Zinc in Mothers of Newborn Infants with Spina Bifida', *Am. J. Clin. Nutr.,* 33 (1980), 2145-2150.
12. Joswigg, T. 'The Effect of Temporary Venous Occlusion on Trace Mineral Concentrations in Plasma', *Am. J. Clin. Nutr.,* 36 (1982), 354-358.
13. Aggett, P.J. and Harris, J.T. 'Current Status of Zinc in Health and Disease States', *Arch. Dis. Childhood,* 54 (1979), 909-917.
14. Gershoff, S., McGandy, R., Nondastuda, A., Pisdyabutra, U. and Tantiwonge, P. 'Trace Minerals in Human and Rat Hair', *Am. J. Clin. Nutr.,* 30 (1977), 868.
15. Greger, J., Higgins, M.M., Abernathy, R, Kirksey, A., DeCorse, M.B. and Baligar, B. 'Nutritional Status of Adolescent Girls in Regard to Zinc, Copper and Iron', *Am. J. Clin. Nutr.,* 31 (1978), 269.
16. Hambidge, K.M., Walravens, P.A., Brown, R.M., Webster, J., White S., Anthony, M. and Roth, R.L. 'Zinc Nutrition of Preschool Children in the Denver Head Start Program', *Am. J. Clin. Nutr.,* 29 (1976), 734.
17. Erten, J., Arcasoy, A., Caudar, A.O., and Cin, S. 'Hair Zinc Levels in Healthy and Malnourished Children', *Am. J. Clin. Nutr.,* 31 (1978), 1172.
18. Laker, M. 'On Determining Trace Element Levels in Man: The Uses of Blood and Hair, *The Lancet,* 31 July 1982, 260-263.
19. Petering, H.G., Yeager, D.W. and Witherup, S.O. 'Trace Element Content of Hair: Cadmium and Lead of Human Hair', *Arch. Environ. Health,* 27 (1973), 327-330.
20. Clemente, G.F. 'Trace Element Composition of Hair in the Italian Population', Conference on Nuclear Activation Techniques in the Life Sciences, Vienna, May 1978.
21. Mertz, W. 'The Essential Trace Elements', *Science,* 213 (1981), 1332-1338.
22. Hambidge, K.M. 'Chromium Nutrition in Man', *Am. J. Clin. Nutr.,* 27 (1974), 505-514.

23. Deeming, S. and Weber, C. 'Hair Analysis of Trace Elements in Human Subjects as Influenced by Age, Sex and Contraceptive Drugs', *Am. J. Clin. Nutr.*, 31 (1978), 1175.
24. Cartwright, G.E. and Wintrobe, M.M. 'Copper Metabolism in Normal Subjects', *Am. J. Clin. Nutr.*, 14 (1964), 224.
25. Wintrobe, M.M., Cartwright, G.E. and Gubler, C.J. 'Studies on the Function and Metabolism of Copper', *J. Nutr.*, 50 (1953) 395.
26. Reinhold, J.G., Krovry, G.A., Ghalambor, M.A. and Bennett, J.C. 'Zinc and Copper Concentrations of Hair of Iranian Villagers', *Am. J. Clin. Nutr.*, 18 (1966), 294.
27. Porter, K.G., McMaster, D., Hemes, M. and Love A.A.G. 'Anaemia and Low Serum Copper During Zinc Therapy', *The Lancet,* 774, 8 October 1977.
28. Salmela, S. and Kilpio, J.O. 'The Effect of Washing Procedures on Trace Element Content of Human Hair', *Anal. Chim. Acta.,* 125 (1981), 131-137.
29. Cranton, E.M., Bland, J.S., Chatt, A., Krakowitz, R. and Wright, J. 'Standardization and Interpretation of Human Hair for Elemental Concentrations', *J. Holistic Health,* 4 (1982), 11-23.
30. Abraham, J.L. 'Trace Elements in Hair', *The Lancet,* 4 September 1982, 554-555.
31. Mahaffey, K., Annest, J.L. and Roberts, J. 'National Estimates of Blood Lead Levels: United States 1976-1980', *N. Engl. J. Med.*, 307 (1982), 573-579.
32. Needleman, H.L. and Barrett, P. 'Deficits in Psychologic and Classroom Performance of Children with Elevated Lead Dentine Levels', *N. Engl. J. Med.*, 300 (1979), 689-695.
33. Cohen, D.J. and Harcherik, D.F. 'Blood Lead in Autistic Children', *The Lancet,* 10 July 1982, 94-95.
34. Kopp, S.J. and Perry, E.F. 'Cardiovascular Actions of Cadmium at Environmental Exposrue Levels', *Science,* 217 (1982), 837-840.
35. Shapiro, I.M., Sumner, A-J., Spitz, L.K. and Bloch, P. 'Neurophysiological and Neuropsychological Function in Mercury-Exposed Dentists', *The Lancet,* 17 July 1982, 61-63.
36. Perl, D.P. 'Intraneuronal Aluminum Accumulation in Amytrophic Lateral Sclerosis and Parkinsonism-dementia in Guam', *Science,* 217 (1982), 1053-1056.

37. Yokel, R.A. 'Hair as an Indicator of Excessive Aluminum Exposure', *Clinical Chemistry,* 28 (1982), 662-665.

Chapter 2

1. Schroeder, H.A. in *Trace Elements and Man,* Devin-Adair Co. Old Greenwich, Connecticut, 1973.
2. B. Schaule and C. Patterson in *Proceedings of an International Experts' Discussion on Lead,* M. Branica, Ed., Pergamon Press, 1979.
3. Schroeder, H.A. and Nelson, A.D. 'Trace Metals in Human Hair', *J. Invest. Dermatology, 58 (1969),* 71
4. McKenzie, J. 'Alteration of Zinc and Copper Concentration of Hair', *Am. J. Clin. Nutr., 31 (1978),* 470.
5. Jacob, R., Klevay, L. and Logan, G. 'Hair as a Biopsy Material: Index of Hepatic Copper', *Am. J. Clin. Nutr., 31 (1973),* 477.
6. Hendrikson, P., Krook, L. and Larssen, B. 'Mechanism of Bone Resorption in a Case of Human Periodontal Disease', *Svensk. Tandl. Tidskn., 62 (1969),* 323.
7. Pate, B. D., Maes.D., *et al.* 'The Variation of Trace Element Concentrations in Single Human Head Hairs', *J. Radioanal. Chem., 15 (1973),* 115.
8. Crounse, R.G. and Van Scott, E.J. 'Changes in Scalp Hair Roots as a Measure of Toxicity from Cancer Chemotherapeutic Drugs', *J. Invest. Derm., 35 (1960),* 83.
9. Katz, S.A. 'The Use of Hair as a Biopsy Material for Trace Elements in the Body', *American Laboratory,* February 1979, 44.
10. R.S. Pekarek, N. Sandstead and R.A. Jacob. 'Abnormal Cellular Immune Responses During Acquired Zinc Deficiency', *Am. J. Clin. Nutr., 32 (1979),* 1466.
11. Klevay, L. 'Hair as a Biopsy Material', *Arch. Intern. Med., 138 (1978),* 1127.
12. Gershoff, S., McGandy, R. and Tantiwonge, P. 'Trace Minerals in Human and Rat Hair', *Am. J. Clin. Nutr., 30 (1977),* 868.
13. Kopito, L.E. and Schwachman, H. 'All This Lead', *Arch. Environ. Health, 29 (1971),* 296.
14. Kennington G.S. 'Soluble and Fixed Elements in Mammalian Hair', *Science, 155 (1971),* 588.
15. Deeming, S. and Weber, C. 'Hair Analysis of Trace Elements in Human Subjects as Influenced by Age, Sex and Contraceptive Drugs', *Am. J. Clin. Nutr., 31 (1978),* 1175.

16. Maugh, T. 'Hair: A Diagnostic Tool to Complement Blood, Serum, and Urine', *Science, 202 (1978),* 1271.

Chapter 3

1. McDonald, G. 'Arsenic in Napoleon's Hair', *Nature, 4798 (1961), 103.*

2. Kopito, L. and Schwachman, H. 'Hair Lead in the Hair of Children with Chronic Lead Exposure', N. Engl. J. Medicine, 276 (1967), 949.

3. Maugh, T. 'Hair: A Diagnostic Tool to Complement Blood, Serum and Urine', *Science, 202 (1978),* 1271.

4. Jervis, R.E., Tiefenbach, B. and Chattopadhyay, A. 'Scalp Hair as Monitor of Pollution Exposure to Environmental Pollutants', *J. Radioanalyst, Chem., 37 (1977),* 751.

5. Chattopadhyay, A. and Jervis, R.E. 'Hair as an Indicator of Multielement Exposure', Eighth Annual Conference on Trace Elements in Environmental Health, Columbia, MO, June 1974.

6. Irulg, L.M., Rocks, P., *et al.* 'Lead and Morbidity: A dose-response Relationship', *The Lancet,* 1 July 1978.

7. Lin-Fu, J. 'Lead Exposure Among Children — A Reassessment', *New Eng. J. Medicine, 300 (1979),* 731.

8. Erickson, J.E., Shirahata, H and Patterson, C. 'Skeletal Concentrations of lead in ancient Peruvians', *N. Eng. J. Medicine.*

9. Chisolm, J.J., Jr. 'Current Status of Lead Exposure and Poisoning in Children', *South. Med. J., 69 (1976),* 529.

10. Settle, D.M. and Patterson, D.C. 'Lead in Albacore: Guide to Lead Pollution in the Americans', *Science, 207 (1980),* 1167.

11. Thomas, H.F. and Elwood, P.C., 'First-flush Water Lead', *The Lancet,* 8 July 1978, 109.

12. Bryce-Smith, D., Mathews, R. and Stephens, R. 'Mental Health Effects of Lead on Children', *Ambio, 7 (1978),* 192.

13. Eisinger, J. and Valeinkas, J. 'Central Nervous System Dysfunction Due to Lead Exposure', *Science, 201 (1978),* 465.

14. Needleman, H., Gunnoe, C., *et al.* 'Deficits in Psychological and Classroom Performance of Children with Elevated Dentine Lead Levels', *N. Engl. J. Medicine, 689 (1979),* 300.

15. Pihl, R.O. and Parkes, M. 'Hair Element content of

Learning-disabled Children', *Science, 198 (1977),* 204.
16. Searle, C.E. and Harnden, D.G. 'Lead in Hair-dye Preparations', *The Lancet,* 17 November 1979, 1070.
17. Marzulli, F.N., Watlington, P.M. and Maibach, H.I. 'Exploratory Skin Penetration Findings Relating to the Use of Lead Acetate Hair Dyes', *Curr. Prob Dermatol., 7(1978),* 196.
18. Kang, H.K., Infante, P.F., Carra, J.S. 'Occupational Lead Exposure and Cancer', *Science, 207 (1980),* 935.
19. Cross, J.D., Dale, I.M., *et al.* 'Methylmercury in Blood of Dentists', *The Lancet,* 5 August 1978, 312.
20. Ellis, K., Vartsky, D., *et al.* 'Cadmium: *In Vivo* Measurement in Smokers and Non-smokers', *Science, 205 (1979),* 323.
21. Durea, G., Mahurkar, S. and Smith, E.C. 'Role of Aluminium in Dialysis Dementia', *Ann. Intern. Med., 88 (1978),* 504.
22. Ward, M.K., Ellis, H.A., *et al.* 'Osteomalacia Dialysis Osteodystrophy: Evidence of Water-borne Aluminium', *The Lancet,* 22 April 1978, 841.
23. Chen, K., Gibbs, C., *et al.* 'Studies on Amyotrophic Lateral Sclerosis' submitted for publication.
24. Mason, K., 'Conspectus of Research on Copper Metabolism and Requirements of Man', *J. Nutrition, 109 (1979),* 1981.
25. Klevay, L.M., 'Hair as a Biopsy Material, Part II. Assessment of Copper Nutriture', *Am. J. Clin. Nutr., 23 (1970),* 1194.
26. Chan, F.I., *et al.* 'Selenium Deficiency and Keshan Disease', *Chinese J. Medicine,* June 1979.

Chapter 4

1. Prasad, A. *Trace Elements in Human Health and Disease,* vols. I and II, Academic Press, New York, 1977.
2. Maugh, T. 'Hair: A Diagnostic Tool to Complement Blood, Serum and Urine', *Science, 202 (1978),* 1171.
3. Corridan, J. 'Head Hair Samples as Indicators of Environmental Pollution', *Environ. Res., 8 (1974),* 12.
4. Yamaguchi, S., Matsumoto, H., *et al.* 'Factors Affecting the Amount of Mercury in Human Scalp Hair', *Am. J. Public Health, 64 (1975),* 484.
5. Hefferren, J. J. 'Usefulness of Chemical Analysis of Head Hair for Exposure to Mercury', *J. Am. Dental Society, 92 (1976),* 1213.

6. Pueschel, S.M. 'Neurological and Psychomotor Functions in Children with an Increased Lead Burden', *Environ. Health Perspectives,* May 1974, 13.
7. Needleman, H.L., Gunnoe, C., Leviton, A., *et al.* 'Deficits in Psychologic and Classroom Performance of Children with Elevated Dentine Lead Levels', *N. Engl. J. Medicine, 300 (1979),* 689.
8. Pihl. R.O. and Parkes, M. 'Hair Element Content in Learning-disabled Children', *Science, 198 (1977),* 204.
9. Kopito, L., Bailey, A., and Schwachman, H. 'Chronic Plumbism in Children. Diagnosis by Hair Analysis', *J. Amer. Med. Assoc., 209 (1969),* 243.
10. Kosuka H. 'Factors Having Influence on the Trace Elements in Hair' *J. Hyg. Chem., 18 (1972),* 7.
11. Creason, J.P., Hinners, T.A., Bumgarner, J.E. and Pinkerton, C. 'Trace Elements in Hair, as Related to Exposure in Metropolitan New York', *Clin. Chem., 21 (1975),* 603.
12. Strain, W.H. and Pories, W.J. 'Zinc Levels of Hair as Tools in Zinc Metabolism', in *Zinc Metabolism,* A. Prasad, ed., C.C. Thomas, Springfield, IL, 1966, 363.
13. Kopito, L., Elian, E. and Schwachman, H. 'Sodium, Potassium, Calcium, and Magnesium in Hair from Neonates with Cystic Fibrosis', *Pediatrics, 49 (1972),* 620.
14. Hambidge, K.M., Cantab, B.C., Rodgerson, D., *et al.* 'Concentration of Chromium in the Hair of Normal Children and Children with Juvenile Diabetes Mellitus', *Diabetes, 17 (1968),* 517.
15. Hambidge, K.M. and Rodgerson, D.O. 'Comparison of Hair Chromium Levels of Multiparous and Parous Women', *Amer. J. Obstet., Gynecol., 103 (1969),* 320.
16. Saner, G., Yuksel, T. and Gurson, C.T. 'Effect of Chromium on Insulin Secretion and Glucose Removal in the New-born', *Am. J. Clin. Nutr., 33 (1980),* 232.
17. Amador, A and Gonzales, A. 'Hair-zinc Concentrations in Diabetic Children', *The Lancet,* 6 December 1975, 1146.
18. Prasad, A. *Trace Elements in Human Health and Disease,* vol. I Academic Press, New York, 1976.
19. Strain, W.H., Steadman, L.T., Lankau, C.A., *et al.* 'Analysis of Zinc Levels in Hair for the Diagnosis of Zinc Deficiency in Man', *J. Lab. Clin. Med., 68 (1967),* 244.
20. Pekarek, R.S., Sandstead, H.H., Jacob, R.A. and

Barcome, D.F. 'Abnormal Cellular Immune Responses During Acquired Zinc Deficiency', *Am. J. Clin. Nutr., 32 (1979),* 1466.

21. Erten, J., Arcasoy, A. and Cavdar, A. 'Hair Zinc in Healthy and Malnourished Children' *Am. J. Clin. Nutr., 31 (1978),* 1172.

22. McKenzie, J.M. 'Content of Zinc in Serum, Urine, Hair and Toenails of New Zealand Adults', *Am. J. Clin. Nutr., 32 (1979),* 570.

23. Bradfield, R.B. and Hambidge, K.M. 'Problems with Hair Zinc as an Indicator of Body Zinc Status', *The Lancet,* 16 February 1980, 363.

24. McKenzie, J.M. 'Alteration of Zinc and Copper Concentration of Hair', *Am. J. Clin. Nutr., 31 (1978),* 470.

25. Nordlund, J. J. Hartley, C. and Fister, J. 'On the Cause of Green Hair', *Arch. Dermatol. 113 (1977),* 1700.

26. Jacob, R.A., Klevay, L.M. and Logan, G.M. 'Hair as an Index of Hepatic Metal in Rats: Copper and Zinc', *Am. J. Clin. Nutr., 31 (1978),* 477.

27. Epstein, O., Boxx, M.B., Lyon, D. and Sherlock, S. 'Hair Copper in Primary Piliary Cirrhosis', *Am. J. Clin. Nutr., 33 (1980),* 965.

28. Rice, E.W. and Goldstein, N.P. 'Copper Content of Hair and Nails in Wilson's Disease', *Metabolism, 10 (1961),* 1085.

29. Deeming, S.B. and Weber, C.W. 'Hair analysis of Trace Minerals in Human Subjects as Influenced by Age, Sex, and Contraceptive Drugs', *Am. J. Clin, Nutr., 31 (1978),* 1175.

30. Bradfield, R.B. and SooHoo, T., 'Effect of Hypochromotrichia on Hair and Zinc During Kwashiorkor', *Am. J. Clin. Nutr., 33 (1980),* 1315.

31. Porter, K-G., Munier, D.M. and Hemes, M.L. 'Anaemia and Low Serum-copper During Zinc Therapy', *The Lancet,* 8 October, 1977, 774.

32. Singh, S. and Bresnan, J-J, 'Menkes-kinky Hair Syndrome and Low Copper Levels in Blood, Hair and Urine', *Am. J. Dis. Child., 125 (1973),* 572.

33. Klevay, L.M. 'Coronary Heart Disease: The Zinc/Copper Hypothesis', *Am. J. Clin. Nutr., 28 (1975),* 764.

34. Spencer, J.S. 'Direct Relationship Between the Body's Copper/Zinc Ratio, Ventricular Premature Beats, and

Sudden Coronary Death', *Am. J. Clin. Nutr., 33 (1980),* 1184.

Chapter 5

1. Galen, R.S. and Gambino,S.R. *Beyond Mortality*. Wiley Medical, New York, 1975.
2. Fries, J. 'Aging, Natural Death and Compression of Morbidity', *New Engl. J. Med., 303 (1980),* 130.
3. Katsumi, T. 'Lead Content of the Hair of Nursing Infants and of their Mothers', *Orient, Journ, Dis. of Infants* (1926).
4. Gordus, A. Privileged communication, U. of Michigan.
5. Gershoff, S., McGandy, R., Nondastuda, A., Pisdyabutra, U. and Tantiwonge, P. 'Trace Minerals in Human and Rat Hair', *Am. J. Clin. Nutr., 30 (1977),* 368.
6. Hafeman, D.G., Sunde, R.A. and Hoekstra, W.G. 'Effect of Dietary Selenium on Erythrocyte and Liver Glutathione Peroxidase in the Rat', *J. Nutr., 104 (1974),* 580.
7. Tus. H., Wah, L. and Peku, R. 'Keshan Disease as it Relates to Selenium Status', *Chinese J. Medicine,* 1979; 'Selenium in the Heart of China', *The Lancet,* 27 October 1979, 890.
8. Spencer, W. 'Body Copper/Zinc, VPB and Sudden Coronary Death', *Am. J. Clin. Nutr., 33 (1980),* 1184.
9. Klevay, L.M. 'Hair as a Biopsy Material II. Assessment of Copper Nutriture', *Am. J. Clin. Nutr., 23 (1970),* 1194.
10. Klevay, L.M. 'Hair as a Biopsy Material', *Arch. Intern. Medicine, 138 (1978),* 1127.
11. Epstein, O., Boxx, A.M., Lyon, T.D. and Sherlock, S. 'Hair Copper in Biliary Cirrhosis', *Am. J. Clin. Nutr., 33 (1980)*.
12. Bradfield, R.B., Cordano, A., Buertt, J. and Graham, G. 'Hair Copper Deficiency', *The Lancet,* 16 August 1980, 344.
13. Bland, J. 'Dietary Calcium, Phosphorus and their Relationship to Bone Formation and Parathyroid Activity', *J. John Bastyr Coll. Natur. Med., 1 (1979),* 3.
14. Bland, J. 'The Dietary Calcium/Phosphorus and Bone Dynamics', submitted for publication.

INDEX